CW00517071

THE LONGEVITY DIET

NEW SERIES

**This Book Includes:
"Intermittent Fasting and
Mediterranean Diet Recipes "**

By Sara Clark and David Clark

INTERMITTENT FASTING

MEDITERRANEAN DIET RECIPES

INTERMITTENT FASTING

55 Recipes For Intermittent Fasting and Healthy Rapid Weight Loss

By David Clark

Introduction:

Intermittent fasting is an example of eating that alternates between times of fasting, normally devouring just water, and non-fasting, generally eating anything a person needs regardless of how stuffing. In the evening time, a person can eat anything he needs for 24 hours and fast for the following 24 hours. This way to deal with weight control is by all accounts upheld by science, just as strict and social practices throughout the planet. Followers of Intermittent fasting guarantee that this training is an approach to turn out to be more careful about food.

Also, an Intermittent fasting diet is somewhat unique from ordinary fasting. This kind of transient fasting doesn't decrease fat-consuming chemicals. Truth be told, logical exploration has shown that the specific inverse occurs and you will begin expanding the movement of fat-consuming catalysts.

An incredible part of Intermittent fasting is that there isn't a lot of exertion included. You can carry on with life, go out to eat, still have your favorite food sources and a periodic treat. The weight loss can be quick or consistent relying upon how you approach it. You can be as severe or loose about your eating as you need and still get more fit. Eating this way is useful for breaking levels as well.

To benefit from Intermittent fasting, you need to fast for at any rate 16 hours. At 16 hours or more, a portion of the stunning advantages of Intermittent fasting kicks in. A simple method to do this is to just skip breakfast each day. This is in reality extremely solid, however, many people will try to disclose to you in any case. By skipping breakfast, you are permitting your body to go into a caloric shortfall, which will enormously build the measure of fat you can consume and the weight you can lose.

Since your body isn't caught up with processing the food you ate, it has the opportunity to zero in on consuming your fat stores for energy and for purifying and detoxifying your body. If you think that it's hard to skip breakfast, you can rather skip a meal, even though I track down this considerably more troublesome.

It truly doesn't make any difference, yet the objective is to broaden the timeframe you spend fasting and loss the measure of time you spend eating. If you have a meal at 6 PM and don't eat until 10 the following morning, you have refrained for 16 hours. Longer is better, however, you can see some beautiful extraordinary changes from every day 16 hours fast.

Chapter: 1 Breakfast

A better smooth fish pasta heat loaded with heaps of vegetables and surprisingly some mysterious beans. The ideal family-accommodating pasta dish that works for babies and adults. There are alternatives to make this gluten-free, lactose-free, or even dairy-free.

Ingredients:

- 1 block chicken stock
- Salt and pepper
- 4 tbsp. Parmesan cheddar
- 2 tsp lemon juice
- 1.25 cups light coconut milk
- 1.5 tbsp. whole meal flour
- 1 tbsp. margarine
- 1 tsp coconut oil
- 425 g canned fish in spring water
- 1/4 cup whole meal breadcrumbs
- 1 cup frozen or tinned peas or corn or veg of decision

Method:

- Preheat oven to 180C.
- Channel fish and spot in a blending bowl.
- Add corn to the bowl and blend well.
- Season with salt and pepper.
- Cook cubed onions in coconut oil until delicate.

- Add onions to fish blend, mix well.
- Add spread to frypan and soften.
- Pour in coconut milk and gradually add the flour, whisking continually to stay away from knots.
- Add 3 tbsp. of the Parmesan cheddar and the lemon juice.
- Disintegrate the stock shape and sprinkle over the top, then add prepared to taste.
- Blend well.
- Pour sauce over the fish combination and mix until very much consolidated.
- Tip into stove confirmation dishes – it is possible that one huge dish, or personal dishes.
- Combine as one whole meal breadcrumb and the leftover Parmesan cheddar and sprinkle over the fish blend.
- Cook in the oven for 25 minutes and afterward grill for a further 5-10 mins until brilliant earthy colored on top.
- Fill in with no guarantees or with steamed greens, pasta, salad, or rice.

2: Sweet Potato & Black Bean Burrito

Sound Sweet Potato and Black Bean Burrito are loaded down with such a lot of goodness. Your number one tortilla or wrap is loaded up with chime pepper, yam, black beans, avocado, and earthy colored rice for a nutritious dish with stunning flavor. These are normally gluten-free (contingent upon the tortilla) veggie-lover burritos that make an astonishing breakfast, lunch, or dinner that is prepared in less than 30 minutes.

Ingredients:

- fine grain ocean salt
- 1 big red onion, cut
- avocado oil (I utilized Primal Kitchen)
- ground chipotle powder
- 4–6 burrito estimated tortillas
- hot sauce or salsa, whenever wanted (I love a tomatillo one with these!!)
- 1 large or 2 little yams, slashed into 1/2" blocks (no compelling reason to strip, simply wash them well!!)
- 1 15-ounce container of black beans, flushed and depleted

Method:

- Preheat stove to 400 F.
- On a material-lined dish, toss red onions and yams with enough avocado oil to cover and a liberal measure of salt and some chipotle powder.
- Prepare for 20-30 minutes, tossing a couple of times, until yams are effectively penetrated with a fork and onions are earthy colored (whatever's cooking excessively, move more to the middle!).
- Add the black beans to the oven and toss to blend.
- Warm tortillas for 30 seconds on each side to make them flexible (this is too essential to keep them from breaking when you try to overlap them!) then do a line of the black bean and yam combination down the center.

- Add hot sauce if utilizing. Crease in sides and roll. As far as I might be concerned, this made 5 burritos, yet it'll shift dependent on the size of your tortillas. Wrap burritos in foil, and hold up!
- To plan, microwave, or utilize a toaster to warm when prepared to eat.

3: Pb and J Overnight Oats

These PB&J Overnight Oats are a definitive make-ahead breakfast that will keep you powered and empowered throughout the day with whole-grain moved oats, chia seeds, peanut butter, and jam. Make your oats with this natively constructed Chia Seed Jam and add your number one fresh organic product. Overnight cereal is a steady staple in my morning meal routine since it is something I can prepare early and I realize will keep me full throughout the morning.

Ingredients:

- 1 cup moved oats
- 1 tablespoon chia seeds
- 1 cup unsweetened almond milk
- 1/2 tablespoon maple syrup
- 1 tablespoon jam or jelly
- 2 tablespoons rich peanut butter

Method:

- Spot all ingredients short the jam in a glass Tupperware and blend.
- Cover and let sit in the cooler for at any rate 2 hours or overnight.
- In the morning, twirl in some jam and appreciate cold.

Porridge is consistently an extraordinary method to begin the day, regardless of whether you're an infant, youngster, or grown-up. My apple and cinnamon porridge is pressed brimming with flavor. You can eat it also, or jazz it up for certain additional ingredients - I like walnut nuts and poppy seeds. My variant is appropriate for vegetarians; however, you can utilize your preferred milk.

Ingredients:

- 2 tbsp. honey
- 1 section moved oats to 2 sections of milk
- 1 apple
- Touch of salt
- Small bunch toasted walnuts, generally chopped

Method:

- Measure the porridge in a little glass then add it to a little sauce container with twice the milk.
- Spot the pan on medium-high heat and bring to the bubble, then turn off the heat.
- Add a touch of salt and mix reliably until you have a thick, velvety blend, this will take about 8-10minutes.
- Mesh the apple and mix half of it into the porridge, then add the cinnamon and honey and blend well.
- Serve the porridge in a bowl then top it with the remainder of the ground apple, some more cinnamon, and honey.
- Sprinkle the toasted walnuts on top, it's a decent option to add some virus milk over the top if you like.

Waffles are a morning meal staple which is as it should be. They're regularly fleecy, sweet, and covered in margarine—who could want anything more? However, in case you're attempting to go for something somewhat better (and would prefer not to hit your daily calorie quantity just after breakfast), choosing appetizing waffles can make breakfast in a hurry quite a lot more stimulating.

Ingredients:

- 1/2 tsp. heating pop
- 3/4 c. chickpea flour
- 1/2 tsp. salt
- 6 huge eggs
- 3/4 c. plain 2% Greek yogurt
- Cucumbers, parsley, yogurt, tomatoes, scallion, and lemon juice, for serving

Method:

- Heat stove to 200°F. Set a wire rack over a rimmed heating sheet and spot it on the stove. Heat waffle iron per bearings.
- In a big bowl, preparing pop, whisk together flour, and salt.
- In a little bowl, whisk together yogurt and eggs.
- Mix wet ingredients into dry ingredients.
- Gently cover waffle iron with nonstick cooking shower and, in clumps, drop ¼ to ½ cup player into each segment of iron and cook until brilliant earthy colored, 4 to 5 minutes.

- Move to the stove and keep warm. Rehash with the leftover player.
- Serve finished off with cucumbers, tomatoes, and scallion threw with olive oil, pepper, salt, and parsley.
- Shower with yogurt blended in with lemon juice.

6: Avocado Quesadillas

Firm quesadillas loaded up with beans, ringer pepper, sautéed onions, avocado, and bunches of cheddar. These avocado black bean quesadillas are filling and make an extraordinary vegan feast as well. They make an extraordinary breakfast and are very filling as well!

Ingredients:

- 4 delicate flour or corn tortillas
- 1 avocado, hollowed, stripped, and cut into pieces
- 4 ounces Manchego cheddar, cut
- 16 canned or jolted jalapeño cuts

Method:

- Get out 1 tortilla on a work surface.
- Spot about a fourth of the cheddar on one half, not very close to the edge so the cheddar won't soften out as it cooks.
- Top cheddar with a fourth of the avocado and four jalapeño cuts.
- Overlap tortilla fifty-fifty over filling to frame a half-circle.
- Heat a grill container or oven over medium heat.
- Slide uncooked quesadilla onto the oven.

- Crunch down with a weight or simply press momentarily with a spatula.
- Cook 1 moment, then flip the quesadilla and flame broil brief more or until cheddar is liquefied.
- Move the quesadilla to a cutting board and cut it into 6 wedges. Serve right away. Rehash with residual ingredients. Makes 24 wedges.

7: Veggie lover Fried 'Fish' Tacos

This recipe for veggie lover fish tacos is loaded with flavor yet, however, so natural to plan! There's no untidy twofold digging of these children, a too basic one bowl fish 'n chips-style hitter is all you need to get incredibly firm vegetarian "fish" bits ideal for ingredient your Baja fish taco wanting. These veggie-lover fish tacos are stunningly presented with an avocado plate of mixed greens and my blackberry margaritas.

Ingredients:

- 2/3 cup water
- 1/2 cup panko breadcrumbs
- 2 teaspoons nori powder (discretionary, for an 'off-putting' taste)
- 1/2 teaspoon salt
- 2 tablespoons lemon juice
- 1/2 cup flour
- 1 (14 ounces) bundle firm or extra firm tofu, depleted and squeezed
- 2 tablespoons soy sauce or tamari
- 1 tablespoon cornstarch

Rich Lime Slaw:

- 2 tablespoons lime juice
- 1/3 cup veggie-lover mayo of decision
- 1/2 teaspoon stew powder
- 1/4 teaspoon ground cumin
- 1/4 teaspoon salt
- 1/2 teaspoon garlic powder
- 4–5 cups finely destroyed cabbage

Method:

- Preheat the stove to 450 degrees F.
- Make the tofu fish sticks: In one bowl, combine as one the soy sauce, lemon juice, and nori powder.
- In another bowl, whisk together the flour and cornstarch, then gradually race in the water to make a play.
- Put the excess breadcrumbs and salt in a third bowl.
- Cut the tofu into finger-like strips, then plunge into the lemon bowl, the flour player, and finely the panko.
- Spot on a lubed preparing sheet and proceed with the remainder of the tofu.
- Heat for 10 minutes, then flip and cook an extra 8 minutes, or until brilliant earthy colored and fresh.
- While the tofu is cooking, whisk together the elements for the slaw in a big bowl: the mayo, lime squeeze, and preparing.
- Taste, adding more flavors/salt depending on the situation.
- Then include the cabbage and throw well, proceeding to throw the cabbage will cover the cabbage and begin to separate it so it's simpler to eat.

- Warm the tortillas, then partition the tofu onto the tortillas and top with slaw.
- Spurt with all the fresher lime juice, whenever wanted, and appreciate!

8: Peach Berry Smoothie

Smoothies are one of my #1-morning meals or evening jolts of energy (so extraordinary when you live someplace blistering!). I love that there are in a real sense unlimited blends and in its single direction my children will cheerfully eat (drink?) their veggies and pack in some extra organic product. This blueberry peach smoothie dairy-free, normally improved and so delightful on account of delicious peaches and blueberries.

Ingredients:

- 1/2 cup almond milk or most loved juice
- 3/4 cup Driscoll's Blueberries
- 1 Tbsp. ground flaxseeds
- 1/2 cup non-fat plain Greek yogurt
- 2 Tablespoons honey
- 1 little peach, generally slashed, or 1/2 cup frozen peaches
- 3 Ounces ice solid shapes (not required if utilizing frozen peaches)

Method:

- Mix blueberries, peach, almond milk, flaxseeds, honey, yogurt, and ice in a blender until pureed and smooth, mixing a few times.
- Serve right away.

9: Green Smoothie at 8 A.M

Beginning your day with a sound Green Breakfast Smoothie is an incredible method to get empowered and feel great. This one is sound and delicious ... a triumphant combo. Drinking this daily smoothie is the thing that assisted me with getting the body and energy to do some unimaginable things. Most smoothies are made with simply foods grown from the ground, which is high in sugar and can cause aggravation. A green smoothie, then again, is made with fruit, plant-based fluid, and verdant greens.

Ingredients:

- 1 huge mango, frozen
- 1 green apple, cored
- 1/2 English cucumber
- 6 little leaves of romaine (or 3 modest bunches of spinach)
- 1/2 lemon, stripped and cultivated
- 2 celery stems
- cold sifted water to mix (around 2 cups)

Method:

- Spot everything into a fast blender and mix until smooth.
- Serve and appreciate right away.

It's another best recipe for irregular fasting referenced in the morning meal list. You can make it easy and within a short time. It's truly tasty and everybody will like it.

Ingredients:

- 1/2 teaspoon salt
- 1 tablespoon ground lemon strip
- 4 boneless skinless chicken bosom parts
- 5 tablespoons fresh lemon juice, isolated
- 1 teaspoon olive oil, partitioned
- 2 tablespoons olive oil, partitioned
- 1 garlic clove, finely cleaved
- 1/4 teaspoon ground black pepper
- 2 garlic cloves, cooked and pounded
- 1/2 teaspoon ocean salt
- 1 medium tomato, cultivated and finely cleaved
- 1/4 teaspoon fresh ground pepper
- 1/4 cup little green pimento-stuffed olives, meagerly cut
- 2 tablespoons fresh basil leaves, finely cut
- 3 tablespoons escapades, washed
- 1 big avocado, split, hollowed, stripped, and finely cleaved

Method:

- In a sealable plastic pack, consolidate chicken and marinade of the lemon strip, 2 tablespoons lemon juice, garlic, 2 tablespoons olive oil, salt, and pepper.
- Seal sack and refrigerate for 30 minutes.

- In a bowl, whisk together the leftover 3 tablespoons lemon juice, staying 1/2 teaspoons olive oil, ocean salt, simmered garlic, and fresh ground pepper.
- Blend in tomato, green olives, escapades, basil, and avocado; put in a safe spot.
- Eliminate chicken from the sack and dispose of marinade.
- Grill over medium-hot coals for 4 to 5 minutes for every side or to the ideal level of doneness.
- Present with Avocado Tapenade.

11: Meal Club Tilapia Parmesan

This is a very basic dish, so several excessively basic side dishes are all you need. These Sautéed Green Beans with Cherry Tomatoes. I would simply keep it simple. I think one normal misinterpretation of this recipe is that it ought to be fresh. "Crusted" in this case simply implies that it is shrouded in Parmesan.

Ingredients:

- black pepper
- 1 scramble hot pepper sauce
- 2 tablespoons lemon juice
- 2 lbs. tilapia filets
- 1/2 cup ground parmesan cheddar
- 3 tablespoons mayonnaise
- 4 tablespoons margarine, room temperature
- 3 tablespoons finely slashed green onions
- 1/4 teaspoon dried basil
- 1/4 teaspoon preparing salt

Method:

- Preheat oven to 350 degrees.
- In a buttered 13-by-9-inch heating dish or jellyroll container, lay filets in a solitary layer.
- Do not stack filets.
- Brush top with juice.
- In a bowl consolidate cheddar, margarine, mayonnaise, onions, and flavors.
- Blend well in with a fork.
- Prepare fish in preheated oven for 10 to 20 minutes or until fish simply begins to piece.
- Spread with cheddar combination and prepare until brilliant earthy colored, about 5minutes.
- Heating time will rely upon the thickness of the fish you use.
- Watch fish intently with the goal that it doesn't overcook.
- Makes 4 servings.
- Note: This fish can likewise be made in an oven.
- Sear 3 to 4 minutes or until practically done.
- Add cheddar and sear another 2 to 3 minutes or until sautéed.

12: Broccoli Dal Curry

Broccoli Curry is a simple and sound sauce or curry dish that can be presented with hot phulkas or steamed rice. This lovely green vegetable is a storage facility of nutrients and minerals. This recipe safeguards every one of the first supplements of broccoli since it doesn't overcook the broccoli florets.

Ingredients:

- 1 – Potato
- 1 - Broccoli
- 1 - Onion
- 1/2 tsp - Ginger and Garlic glue
- 1/4 cup - Cut Corn
- 1/2 tsp - Dhania Jeera powder
- 1/2 tsp - Urad dal
- Salt and Red Chili powder to taste
- 1 squeeze - Turmeric powder
- 1/2 tsp - Mustard seeds
- 4 tsp - Oil

Method:

- Cut the broccoli into little pieces and cook in the microwave for 6 minutes.
- Heat oil in a container and add urad dal, mustard seeds and fry them to a brilliant brown tone.
- Cleave the onion and potato into pieces, add it to the above blend and fry till the potato is bubbled.
- Add to the abovementioned, ginger and garlic glue, dhania and jeera powder, a little turmeric powder, and if you need 1/2 tsp garam masala.
- Add the cooked broccoli pieces alongside slicing corn and salt to taste and red stew powder, and cook it for 5 minutes.
- Your broccoli curry is fit to be presented with one or the other rice or chapatti.

13: Pie Maker Zucchini Slice Muffins

Here is another best recipe for your morning meal. You can undoubtedly make this recipe at your home. It's an astonishing recipe that everybody will very much want to have.

Ingredients:

- 200g yam, stripped, coarsely ground
- 80ml (1/3 cup) extra virgin olive oil
- 2 medium zucchini (about 300g), managed, coarsely ground
- 5 eggs, delicately whisked
- 150g (1 cup) self-rising flour
- 100g (1 cup) Perfect Italiano Perfect Bakes cheddar (mozzarella, cheddar, and parmesan)

Method:

- Heat 1 tablespoon of the oil in a medium non-stick oven over medium-high heat.
- Add the yam and cook, mixing periodically, for 5 minutes or until mollified. Move to a big bowl.
- Add the zucchini, flour, cheddar, egg, and remaining oil.
- Season well and mix to join.
- Preheat the pie producer.
- Fill the pie producer openings with a yam blend.
- Close, cook for 8 minutes.
- Rehash with the excess blend.
- Serve warm or cold.

14: Simmered Broccoli with Lemon-Garlic and Toasted Pine Nuts

So natural thus great. Simmered broccoli with lemon zing, pine nuts, and a sprinkle of Parmesan, on the table in minutes with a little prep work. You'll cherish how the fresh, dynamic broccoli gets punched up with fiery stew chips and a solid hit of lemon juice, in addition to the stunning, rich kind of toasted pine nuts.

Ingredients:

- 2 tablespoons olive oil
- 1-pound broccoli florets
- 2 tablespoons unsalted spread
- 1 teaspoon minced garlic
- Salt and freshly ground black pepper
- 1/2 teaspoon ground lemon zing
- 2 tablespoons pine nuts, toasted
- 1 to 2 tablespoons fresh lemon juice

Method:

- Preheat oven to 500°F.
- In a big bowl, throw the broccoli with the oil and salt, and pepper to taste.
- Mastermind the florets in a solitary layer on a preparing sheet and meal, turning once, for 12 minutes, or until simply delicate.
- In the meantime, in a little pot, soften the spread over medium heat.
- Add the garlic and lemon zing and heat, blending, for around 1 moment.
- Let cool somewhat and mix in the lemon juice.
- Spot the broccoli in a serving bowl, pour the lemon margarine over it and throw to cover.
- Dissipate the toasted pine nuts over the top and serve.

Hard-bubbled eggs are an extraordinary food to have available as their uses are so adaptable. In addition to the fact that they are too delectable all alone, yet they're incredible in sandwiches, cleaved up on a salad, and the establishment for all devilled eggs. The secret to incredible hard-bubbled eggs isn't over-cooking them, which can leave a dim ring around the yolk and make their surface somewhat rubbery.

Ingredients:

- 1 tbsp. Sea salt
- 4 cups Water (or enough to cover eggs in the oven)
- 8 big Egg (or any number you need)
- 1 tbsp. Apple juice vinegar (or white if not paleo)

Method:

- Spot your crude eggs in a medium pan and cover with at least 2 creeps of cold water.
- Add 1 tablespoon of salt.
- Spot the dish over high heat until it arrives at a bubble.
- Mood killer heat, cover, and let it sit for 13 minutes.
- After precisely 13 minutes, eliminate the eggs from the dish and spot them in an ice-water shower and let them cool for five minutes.
- Cautiously break the eggs shells (ensuring most of the shell is broken).
- Delicately start eliminating the shells. The ice-water shower will "stun" the film in the middle of the egg-white and the eggshell, releasing the shell and permitting you to strip it off in almost one piece.

- Depending on the situation, you can plunge the egg (as you are stripping it) all through the water to eliminate any bits of the shell.
- Serve promptly, use in a recipe, or store in your fridge for three days.

16: Turkish Egg Breakfast

Turkish eggs recipe creates the ideal breakfast. Turkish Menemen Recipe is an incredibly delectable breakfast recipe. Summer tomatoes and green peppers consolidate with eggs in a container to simplify this, fast, and very yummy supper.

Ingredients:

- 2 tsp lemon juice
- 1 garlic clove, squashed
- 200g/7oz Greek-style plain yogurt
- 1 tsp ocean salt pieces
- 2 tbsp. unsalted spread
- 1 tsp Aleppo pepper
- 1 tbsp. extra virgin olive oil
- 2 huge free-roaming eggs, ice chest cold
- thick sourdough toast, to serve
- barely any fronds fresh dill, cleaved

Method:

- Top a pan off to 4cm/1½in profound with water and bring to the bubble.
- Spot the yogurt into a heatproof bowl sufficiently big to sit over the oven and mix in the garlic and salt.
- Spot the bowl over the oven, ensuring the base doesn't contact the water.

- Mix until it arrives at the internal heat level and has the consistency of softly whipped twofold cream.
- Mood killer the heat, leaving the bowl over the dish.
- Dissolve the spread tenderly in a different little pan until it is simply starting to turn hazelnut-earthy colored.
- Turn the heat off, then mix in the oil, trailed by the Aleppo pepper, and put in a safe spot.
- Fill a wide, lidded pot with 4cm/1½in water and spot over medium heat. Line a big plate with kitchen paper.
- Break the initial egg into a little fine-network sifter suspended over a little bowl, then lift and twirl delicately for around 30 seconds, giving the watery piece of the white trickle access to the bowl; dispose of.
- Delicately tip the egg into a little cup or ramekin and pour 1 teaspoon of lemon juice onto it, focusing on the white. Rehash with the subsequent egg.
- At the point when the poaching water is simply beginning to stew, tenderly slide in the eggs, one on each side of the oven.
- Turn the heat directly down so there is no development in the water, and poach the eggs for 3–4 minutes, until the whites are set and the yolks still runny.
- Move the eggs to the lined plate utilizing an opened spoon.
- Separation the warm, rich yogurt between two shallow dishes, top each with a poached egg, pour over the peppery spread, dissipate the slashed dill on top and eat with the toast.

Simple to make, with simple ingredients, these clammy vegetarian banana biscuits are a pleasant base for fruit, nuts, and even chocolate chips. Blend and match your number one extra items to make your form utilizing our recipe as a format. Eat these biscuits warm with vegetarian margarine and natural product for breakfast, with nut spread for a protein-stuffed bite, or with a scoop of veggie lover frozen yogurt for a simple and tasty pastry.

Ingredients:

- 1 cup oats
- 1 tsp. vanilla concentrate
- 3 bananas
- 3 tbsp. maple syrup
- 1 cup coconut milk
- 1 tsp. heating pop
- 2 tsp. heating powder
- ½ cup slashed walnuts
- 2 tbsp. chipped or destroyed coconut
- 1 ¼ cups whole wheat flour + ¼ cup coconut flour

Method:

- Preheat oven to 350.
- Line 12 biscuit tins with papers. In a medium blending bowl, blend oats, flour(s), heating pop, and preparing powder.
- In a different bowl, pound bananas well with a fork or potato masher.
- Add vanilla, maple syrup, and coconut milk.

- Whisk everything together well, and afterward adds to dry ingredients. Blend until just mixed.
- Overlay in walnuts.
- A split blend between biscuit tins.
- Sprinkle biscuit tops with coconut.
- Prepare 23-27 minutes, or until tops simply start to firm and coconut starts to brown.

Chapter: 2 Lunch

18: Turmeric Tofu Scramble

Tofu can be scary, yet this flexible plant protein takes on whatever flavor you give it. With each chomp of this exquisite scramble recipe, you'll feel better and stimulated. This morning meal will likewise help deal with your glucose levels. This turmeric tofu scramble is made with delightful, supplement-pressed flavors and is an amazing plant-based option in contrast to your commonplace egg-driven lunch.

Ingredients:

- 1 teaspoon turmeric powder
- 2 tablespoons healthful yeast (optional)
- 1/4 teaspoon cayenne pepper
- freshly ground black pepper (MUST)
- 2 tablespoons non-dairy milk or Veganaise
- grapeseed oil for cooking
- 1/2 teaspoon fine ocean salt
- 1/2 bundle (15 oz.) natural firm tofu (grew is extraordinary as well)

Method:

- Channel the tofu from the water and break the tofu into little scraps.
- Add the nourishing yeast, turmeric, pepper, salt, and milk, and mix well.
- Heat nonstick skillet on a low heat, then add oil.
- Add the tofu into the skillet and cook for around 3-4 minutes mixing sporadically.
- Add the child spinach and cover with a top to permit the heat to steam the spinach.
- Turn the heat off when you do this and reveal and two or multiple times more.
- Serve hot with cherry tomatoes and avocado toast. (red peppers or different veggies likewise work incredibly, however, tomatoes are a lot speedier to cook and the concentration here is 5 minutes.

19: Shredded Brussels Sprouts with Bacon and Onions

Shredded Brussels sprouts are my #1 fresh dish, truly give me a fork. It's a side dish that meets up super-quick. Each chomp is stacked with flavor, toss with garlic, and finished off with a firm, smoky bacon. It makes the whole cycle a lot simpler and truly shreds the fledglings into a flawless knot of green. You can likewise utilize a sharp blade and get the cuts as slim as could be expected.

Ingredients:

- 4 cups chicken stock or low-sodium stock
- Coarse salt and freshly ground pepper
- 1 Spanish onion, daintily cut
- 8 garlic cloves, split the long way
- 4 pounds Brussels sprouts, managed

- 1/2 pound thickly cut lean bacon, cut across into flimsy strips
- Sugar (optional)

Method:

- In a big, profound skillet, cook the bacon over tolerably high heat until caramelized, around 8 minutes.
- Add the onion and garlic, reduce the heat to direct, and cook, mixing, until relaxed, around 5 minutes.
- Add the stock, season with salt and pepper and a spot of sugar, and cook until the fluid has reduced to 1 cup, around 12 minutes.
- Then, in a large pot of bubbling salted water, whiten the Brussels sprouts until scarcely delicate, around 3 minutes.
- Add the fledglings to the skillet. Stew delicately over moderate heat, mixing every so often, until delicate all through, around 10 minutes; season with salt and pepper.
- Utilizing an opened spoon, move to a bowl.
- Heat the fluid in the skillet over tolerably high heat until reduced to 1/2 cup. Pour the sauce over the Brussels fledglings and serve.

20: Vegan Coconut Kefir Banana Muffins

These biscuits taste natural and consoling, given their feathery, banana-mixed internal parts. They're also fun and tropical, because of the Shredded coconut you'll discover within and on the biscuit tops. A little lemon zing unites every one of the flavors.

These biscuits are improved with essentially ready bananas, with simply a trace of coconut palm sugar (or brown sugar). If you don't have these elective flours available, simply supplant them with wheat or gluten-free flour of your decision. With just 10 ingredients, these sound, plant-based biscuits are not difficult to heat up, and they will be a certain fire hit with the whole family.

Ingredients:

- ½ cup virgin coconut oil, dissolved
- ¼ cup honey
- 1 ½ teaspoon preparing powder
- ¼ teaspoon fine ocean salt
- ½ cup white whole wheat flour or ordinary whole wheat flour
- ¾ cup unsweetened Shredded coconut, isolated
- 1 tablespoon turbinado (crude) sugar
- ½ teaspoon lemon zing (the zing from about ½ medium lemon)
- 1 cup squashed ready banana (from around 3 bananas)
- 1 big egg, ideally at room temperature
- 1 teaspoon vanilla concentrate
- ¾ cup whole wheat baked good flour or white/standard whole wheat flour

Method:

- Preheat stove to 375 degrees Fahrenheit. If important, oil every one of the 12 cups of your biscuit tin with spread or biscuit liners (my dish is non-stick and didn't need any oil).

- In a medium bowl, whisk together the flours, salt, heating powder, and lemon zing. Mix in ½ cup of the shredded coconut.
- In a different, medium bowl, whisk together the pounded banana, honey, coconut oil, egg, and vanilla.
- Empty the wet ingredients into the dry ingredients and mix until just consolidated.
- Separation the player uniformly between the biscuit cups (a meager ¼ cup hitter every), then sprinkle the biscuit tops with the excess ¼ cup Shredded coconut.
- Sprinkle the tops with crude sugar.
- Prepare for around 17 to 20 minutes, until a toothpick embedded into the middle, tells the truth.
- Move biscuits to a cooling rack and let them cool.

21: Avocado Ricotta Power Toast

This avocado toast gets a novel turn with extra garnishes of lemon ricotta, kale microgreens, and a sprinkle of all that bagel zest. This ricotta avocado toast is uncommonly acceptable, getting its splendid, fresh taste from the lemony ricotta. The pillowy ricotta shapes the base for the avocado which gets finished off with a runny egg for additional flavor. Polished off with a sprinkling of fragile microgreens and a sprinkle of all that bagel zest, this toast shines a different light on the words simple, workday breakfast.

Ingredients:

- 4 eggs
- 6 tablespoons ricotta cheddar
- 3 avocados, crushed
- 4 tablespoons harissa

- 4 cups of whole wheat, toasted
- 1/4 cup cut green onions
- 1 teaspoon white vinegar

Method:

- Fill a big skillet around 1/2″ loaded with water.
- Heat to the point of boiling.
- Add bread to toaster oven and toast until somewhat sautéed.
- Eliminate and let sit.
- Add a sprinkle of white vinegar to the bubbling water (around 1 teaspoon).
- Quickly include 4 eggs separating them. Cover.
- Turn burners off.
- Leave eggs covered with the heat off for 4-5 minutes.
- Meanwhile, add 1/2 tablespoons of ricotta to each piece of toast, just as 1/4 cup of squashed avocado, and 1 tablespoon of harissa.
- When eggs poached.
- Delicately eliminate from water (make certain to empty any fluid of the skillet) and spot on top of amassed toast.
- Embellishment with green onions.
- Serve!

22: Vegan Lentil Burgers

Burgers will consistently be one of my #1 food varieties! These Completely Vegan Lentil Burgers permit you to appreciate this exemplary fave yet in a MUCH better manner! Every burger contains such a lot of plant-based goodness; your body will much be obliged.

These fiery Vegan Lentil Burgers are made with split red lentils and are finished off with the most delectable rich vegetarian avocado sauce. Prepared in less than 20 minutes, these lentil patties are extraordinary as burgers, lettuce wraps, or in a salad.

Ingredients:

- 1 onion, slashed
- ½ pound (227 g) of mushrooms, freshly cut
- 2 tablespoons (30 mL) of vegetable oil
- 2 cups (500 mL) of cooked lentils
- 4 cloves of garlic, freshly slashed
- 1 cup (250 mL) of bread morsels
- 2 tablespoons (30 mL) of dried thyme
- ½ cup (125 mL) of nut or almond margarine
- ¼ cup (60 mL) of chia seeds
- 2 tablespoons (30 mL) of miso glue
- 2 tablespoons (30 mL) of soy sauce
- 2 cups (500 mL) of yam, ground

Method:

- Sprinkle the oil into your skillet over medium-high heat.
- Toss in the mushrooms, onion, and garlic, and sauté until they become brown and tasty around 10 minutes. Move the mix to your food processor.
- Add every one of the excess ingredients except the ground yam. Puree the combination until everything is easily joined.

- Move the combination to a mixing bowl and mix in the yam by hand so it doesn't separate in the machine.
- Rest the combination for ten minutes, giving the chia seeds time to do something amazing.
- Utilizing your hands, shape the mix into equally framed patties.
- They might be cooked promptly, refrigerated for a few days, or frozen for a month.
- When the time has come to cook you have heaps of alternatives for these burgers.
- You may broil them in a daintily oiled sauté skillet on your burner, singe them on your iron, barbecue, or BBQ, or even prepare in your broiler at 400°F (200°C) for 15 to 20 minutes.
- Whatever method you pick, remember that these burgers brown moderately rapidly so medium-high heat will permit the focuses to keep up while the outsides cook.

23: Baked Mahi Mahi

It's an incredible, more affordable option in contrast to halibut, and can be barbecued, cooked, or even singed. Yet, one of our number one different ways to set it up is to just dish burn it, which lets the flavors and flaky surface sparkle. Singing it in a skillet also allows you to make a rich, lemony sauce to shower everywhere on the fish. All you need to finish this simple fish meal is a green salad or vegetable, and possibly some bread or rice to sop up all that delectable sauce. Here's the simplest method to cook mahi mahi.

Ingredients:

- ¼ tsp salt
- ¾ cup cream
- ¼ tsp pepper
- ½ cup raspberry juice
- ¼ cup balsamic vinegar
- 1 tbsp. spread
- 6-piece medium size mahi-mahi

Method:

- Spread 1 tablespoon of margarine on 6 bits of medium-sized mahi-mahi and sprinkle it with 1/4 teaspoon every one of pepper and salt.
- Orchestrate the fishes on a lubed heating dish. Pour 3/4 cup of cream and 1/4 cup of Balsamic vinegar over the fish.
- Cover the heating dish with material paper and spot it inside a broiler that has been preheated to 450 degrees Fahrenheit. Cook for 12 minutes.

24: Grass-Fed Burgers

If you've changed to grass-took care of meat, you likely realize that it's liberated from chemicals and lower in fat, and higher in some significant supplements than ordinary grain-took care of hamburger. If you bought it simply from a limited-scale farmer, you may likewise be aware of subtleties like the cows' variety and age.

Ingredients:

- 4 teaspoons fit salt
- 2 lbs. Belcampo ground hamburger
- 4 Slices provolone cheddar

- 8 Slices cooked bacon
- 4 Brioche burger buns
- 4 Slices tomato and other burger garnishes (pickles, red onion)

Method:

- Separation 2 lbs. grass-took care of hamburger into four segments.
- To not exhaust the meat, eliminate it from the bundle and simply shape it into burger patties around 5" across – don't massage the meat.
- Sprinkle every burger with one teaspoon Kosher salt partitioned one half on each side
- Preheat barbecue on high
- Cook for 3 minutes on each side for Medium Rare, 4 minutes on each side for Medium. Eliminate from heat when inner temp arrives at 125F.
- Spot cheddar on the burger after the main flip
- Eliminate from the flame broil and spot on a bun with garnish and cooked Bacon

25: Cinnamon Roll Fat Bombs

The cinnamon fat bombs are made keto-accommodating by keeping the ingredients low carb and high fat, and the cream cheddar icing is amazingly acceptable. This is genuinely a high-fat keto bite that is amazing. Here's a recipe for making cinnamon simply move fat bombs.

Ingredients:

- ½ cup almond flour
- ½ cup unsalted margarine, at room temperature

- 1 tsp ground cinnamon
- 3 ½ tbsp. granulated Stevia or another granulated sugar to taste
- For cream cheddar icing:
- ½ tsp vanilla concentrate
- 3 tbsp. cream cheddar
- 1 ½ tbsp. substantial cream
- 1 ½ tbsp. granulated Stevia or another granulated low carb sugar to taste

Method:

- In a bowl place the spread and granulated Stevia and utilizing an electric mixer beat on medium speed until mixed.
- Add the almond flour and cinnamon and beat to consolidate.
- Cover the batter and refrigerate for 30 minutes or until adequately hard to frame balls.
- Free the mixture once again from the fridge and fold into balls around 1 tablespoon in size.
- Freeze the balls for 20 minutes.
- To make the icing, in a microwave-safe bowl join every one of the ingredients.
- Microwave on high for 20 seconds.
- Eliminate from the microwave and mix.
- Shower the icing over the balls.
- Keep the balls in a water/airproof holder in the fridge until prepared to serve.

26: Cauliflower Popcorn

This low-carb cauliflower popcorn is perhaps the yummiest (and generally fun!) approach to eat cauliflower. No spongy business here! With its wonderfully firm covering, this dish is a hit with the whole family, if they are watching their carbs. Functions admirably as finger food, as an hors d'oeuvre, or as a side dish.

Ingredients:

- 1 cup (75g) panko breadcrumbs

- 1 teaspoon smoked paprika
- 1 Coles Australian Free Range Egg, delicately whisked
- 2 teaspoons coarsely chopped thyme twigs
- 1 cauliflower, cut into little florets
- 1/2 cup (40g) finely ground parmesan

Method:

- Preheat stove to 200°C. Line a preparing plate with heating paper.
- Cook the cauliflower in a big pot of bubbling water for 5 mins or until simply delicate. Channel well.
- Move to a big bowl. Mix in the egg.
- Consolidate the breadcrumbs, parmesan, paprika, and thyme in a big bowl. Add the cauliflower mix and toss to join.
- Mastermind the mix in a solitary layer over the lined plate. Shower well with olive oil splash. Season.

27: Best Baked Potato

This heated potato recipe is pretty much as a clear record as it gets. Don't hesitate to add different flavors to the salt-and-pepper mix, like cumin or smoked paprika, and get done with whatever cheddar you like. In case you're utilizing little potatoes, you can slice them down the middle or if they're minuscule, you can simply give them a little jab with a fork or blade before preparing to permit the steam to getaway.

Ingredients:

- 1/4 cup olive oil
- 1 tablespoon salt

- 4 big Russet potatoes

Method:

- Preheat the stove to 425 degrees.
- Wash and dry the potatoes.
- Puncture the potato 2-3 times with a fork
- Rub oil everywhere on the potatoes (or pick one of the different alternatives above to rub outwardly).
- Rub salt everywhere on the potatoes. We incline toward coarse ocean salt or pink Himalayan salt.
- Spot the potatoes on a preparing sheet and heat for around 45 minutes.
- The specific preparing time will rely upon how big the potatoes are. The potato ought to be delicate inside if you stick a fork into it.
- Present with spread, chives, cheddar, sharp cream, and the entirety of your #1 garnishes!

28: Crispy Cauliflower Pizza Crust

Cauliflower Pizza Crust is extremely popular however if you don't make it effectively, it tends to be a spongy disillusionment. The objective is to have a decent firm hull, not a limp, soft wreck. After much experimentation, we at last sorted out the key to the whole fresh Cauliflower Pizza Crust.

This cauliflower pizza outside layer recipe utilizes basic ingredients with the goal that you can the entirety of the tasty garnishes you like. It's low carb, gluten-free, without grain, and pressing the flavor. This is what you'll have to make it:

Ingredients:

- 2 pounds' cauliflower florets riced

- 1 egg beaten
- 1 teaspoon dried oregano
- 1/4 teaspoon Himalayan salt
- 1/2 cup ground mozzarella cheddar or Parmesan cheddar

Method:

- Preheat stove to 400 degrees F.
- Heartbeat bunches of crude cauliflower florets in a food processor, until a rice-like surface, is accomplished. However, don't over-cycle or cream it.
- Microwave the cauliflower rice for around 1 moment or until delicate. Or heat it: In a large pot, load up with about an inch of water, and heat it to the point of boiling.
- Add the cauliflower "rice" and cover. Cook around 4-5 minutes. After the cauliflower is cooked, channel it into a fine sifter or over cheesecloth.
- On your counter over a towel, spread out a fine-network cheesecloth.
- Pour the mix on the cheesecloth and utilizing the cheesecloth, assemble and press out any additional dampness into the sink.
- Pat much more dampness out by tapping again with the towel. Ensure all the water is taken out by crushing out on the towel.
- Whenever dampness is taken out, move "rice" to a large mixing bowl. Add beaten egg, cheddar, oregano, and salt. You may have to utilize your hands to mix.

- Press the mixture out onto a heating sheet fixed with material paper.
- Utilizing hands press level and crush in the sides to frame a shape at ⅓ inch high. Make marginally higher on the sides.
- Heat 35-40 minutes at 400 degrees F or until the outside layer is firm and amazing brown.
- Eliminate from broiler and add garnishes.
- Heat an extra 5-10 minutes until cheddar is hot and effervescent. Serve right away.

29: Almond Apple Spice Muffins

These paleo apple biscuits are so fast and simple to assemble thus great! Heat them toward the end of the week and freeze for in and out morning meals during the week. They're gluten-free and without grain with a sans dairy alternative.

Ingredients:

- 1 teaspoon allspice
- 1 teaspoon cloves
- 2 cups almond meal
- 4 eggs
- 1 cup unsweetened fruit purée
- 5 scoops of vanilla protein powder
- 1/2 stick margarine
- 1 tablespoon cinnamon

Method:

- Preheat the broiler to 350 degrees. Liquefy margarine in the microwave (~30 seconds on low heat).
- Completely mix every one of the ingredients in a bowl.

- Splash biscuit tin with non-stick cooking shower or use cupcake liners.
- Empty mix into biscuit tins, make a point, not to overload (~3/4 full); this should make 12 biscuits (2 biscuit plate).
- Spot one plate in the broiler and cook for 12 minutes.
- Make a point not to overcook as the biscuits will turn out to be extremely dry.
- When cooked, eliminate from the broiler and cook the second biscuit plate.

30: Healthy Mexican Fried Rice

This Mexican singed rice recipe is also an extraordinary method to rapidly make a side dish utilizing precooked rice from a clump cooking meeting or extra rice. The way to making incredible singed rice is utilizing cooked, cold rice. When I make any kind of singed rice recipe, I like to clump cook rice the other day and refrigerate it short-term so it gets quite cold. Cooked rice also freezes well if you needed to make a bigger group and freeze it in the sums you need for this and other rice plans.

Ingredients:

- 2 teaspoons olive oil
- 100 grams (1/2 cup) brown rice
- 1 little yellow onion, sliced
- 1 garlic clove, squashed
- 1 little bean stew pepper, deseeded and chopped
- 1 teaspoon Mexican stew powder
- 1/2 can corn portions
- 1/2 can black beans, washed

- 1 tablespoon fresh lime juice
- 100-gram grape tomatoes, chopped
- Fresh coriander, to serve
- Lime wedges, to serve
- 60-gram feta disintegrated
- 1/4 little red onion, finely slashed
- 1/2 little avocado, quartered and cut

Method:

- Cook the rice in a large pan of bubbling water for 25 minutes or until delicate.
- Channel well, then spread onto a large plate and spot into the ice chest, uncovered, for at any rate 60 minutes.
- Heat the oil in a big griddle over medium heat.
- Add the yellow onion and stew pepper, and cook for five minutes or until delicate. Add the garlic and bean stew powder.
- Proceed to cook and mix for 30 seconds or until fragrant.
- Add the rice and cook, mixing, for two minutes until softly seared and all around joined with the onion mix.
- Add the beans and corn and keep cooking, mixing regularly, until warmed through. Pour lime squeeze over and toss to consolidate.
- Consolidate the tomatoes and red onion and season to taste.
- Split the rice mix between serving bowls and top with the tomato combination, feta, avocado, coriander, and lime wedges.

31: Turkey Tacos

Here is another best recipe for your lunch. This recipe has a couple of stunts at its disposal to ensure each chomp is delicious and completely prepared. Coming to tortillas close to you in around 15 minutes.

Ingredients:

- 8 taco shells
- 1 tablespoon olive oil
- 1-pound ground turkey
- 1 little yellow onion, slashed
- ½ teaspoon bean stew powder
- Salt
- 1 ½ cups (6 ounces) shredded Cheddar
- 1 little head of romaine lettuce, Shredded
- 1 beefsteak tomato, cubed

Method:

- Heat the oil in a medium heat.
- Add the onion and cook, mixing, until marginally delicate, around 4 minutes.
- Add the turkey and cook, disintegrating with the rear of a spoon, until no hint of pink remaining parts, 5 to 7 minutes.
- Mix in the bean stew powder and ½ teaspoon salt.
- Spoon the filling into the taco shells and top with lettuce, Cheddar, and tomato.

Making hand-crafted bolognese sauce is simpler than you'd suspect! This healthy bolognese is a delectable, flavorful dish that you can make without any preparation in just 25 minutes.

Ingredients:

- 2 garlic cloves, stripped and finely sliced
- 1 tsp light olive oil
- 1 medium onion, finely sliced
- 1 medium courgette, finely cubed
- 1 celery sticks, finely sliced
- 600ml meat stock
- 400g turkey mince
- 1 big carrot, ground
- 2 sound leaves
- 300g whole-wheat spaghetti
- 150ml red wine (optional)
- 400g tin sliced tomatoes
- Parmesan shavings, to serve
- basil leaves, to serve

Method:

- Heat the oil in a big, non-stick, weighty lined pan.
- Add the onion, celery, and 2 tablespoons water and fry for 5 minutes or until the vegetables have mellowed.
- Add the courgette and fry for another 2-3 minutes.
- Add the mince and garlic and fry for another 3-4 minutes, mixing now and again or until the mince has separated and is beginning to brown. Mix well.

- Add the ground carrot and 150ml of the hamburger stock or red wine, whenever liked, and stew for 3-4 minutes.
- Then add the tinned tomatoes, 450ml hamburger stock, and the narrows leaves and bring them to the heat.
- Cover with a top, turn down the heat to medium-low, and leave to stew for 45 minutes, mixing once in a while.
- Eliminate the cover and cook for another 10-15 minutes, or until the fluid has reduced and thickened to wanted consistency.
- Cook the spaghetti as per parcel directions, channel, and split between 6 plates. Spot a spoonful of Bolognese on top of each plate, dissipate with basil leaves and Parmesan shavings.

33: Trail Mix

The trail mix nibble recipe I am showing you today is exceptionally healthy since it is wealthy in cancer prevention agents. As you may know, cell reinforcements advance great wellbeing as they help stay away from infections. All the more explicitly, cancer prevention agents help hinder the oxidation of cells in our body.

When cells oxidize, they create free extremists, which are otherwise called cell bi-items. It is protected to have a sensible measure of these free revolutionaries in the body. Notwithstanding, when the free revolutionaries are in abundance, they can unleash ruin on our organic entity's cell mechanical assembly.

Ingredients:

- Cheerios
- Wheat, corn, or rice Chex cereal
- Low-fat popcorn
- Low-fat granola cereal bunches
- Low-fat sesame seeds
- Unsalted pretzel winds or sticks
- Unsalted sunflower seeds (shelled)
- Sans sugar chocolate chips or M&Ms
- Soy nuts
- Unsalted scaled-down rice cakes

Method:

- You can likewise buy low sugar or sans sugar dried fruit at different wellbeing food stores.
- Likewise, one of the most reduced sugar-dried fruits is apple.
- Figs are another healthy decision.
- If you should utilize high glossed-over treats, use them with some restraint.
- While setting up these treats, you can toss them in close Ziploc baggies that are not difficult to bring on picnics, strolls, or any place you go.

34: Weight Watchers Berry Crisp

This Weight Watchers Berry Crisp is a delightful and simple sweet you don't need to feel remorseful about enjoying. This fast, 5-ingredient treat hits every one of the spots of those old top choices yet with way fewer calories. The recipe is made with fresh berries and improved with a dash of brown sugar and a trace of cinnamon. It's done off with a fresh ingredient made of low-fat granola.

Ingredients:

- 1½ cups raspberries
- 1½ cups fresh blackberries
- 1½ cups blueberries
- ¾ cup generally useful flour
- ¼ cup sugar
- ½ cup amazing brown sugar, stuffed
- ¾ cup moved oats
- ½ teaspoon cinnamon
- Fat-free frozen vanilla yogurt, optional
- ½ cup reduced-fat margarine, cold
- Gently whipped cream, optional

Method:

- Preheat broiler to 350 degrees
- In a medium bowl utilizing an elastic spatula, delicately toss together the blackberries, raspberries, blueberries, and white sugar; put in a safe spot
- In a different medium bowl, join flour, oats, brown sugar, and cinnamon. Add the margarine in pieces and cautiously mix while keeping brittle.
- Coat 6 (3 ½-inch) ramekins with a cooking splash, see prep tip. Split the sugared berries between them.
- Separation and sprinkle equitably absurd the disintegrate mix, about ⅓ cup for each.
- Line a preparing sheet with material paper or foil. Spot the 6 ramekin cups on the skillet.
- Prepare for around 40 minutes until amazing brown. Top with a little whipped cream or frozen yogurt, whenever wanted.

San Choy Bau is one of those dishes my children continue to request over and over. It's an incredible one for outdoors in the light of the fact that the ingredients store effectively (clam sauce ought to be kept in the refrigerator), and you just need one skillet. A similar sum functions as a starter for a large gathering (diamond lettuce goes home better for this) – or feed the family as a simple without carb lunch.

Ingredients:

- 500g pork mince
- 1 tablespoon ground ginger
- 1/4 cup clam sauce
- 2 garlic cloves, finely slashed
- 1 tablespoon nut oil
- 2 tablespoons kecap manis
- 2 teaspoons lime juice
- 1/2 tablespoon caster sugar
- 1 teaspoon sesame oil
- coriander leaves
- 1 little chunk of ice lettuce
- salted carrots
- singed shallots
- 1/4 cup slashed peanuts, gently cooked with salt

Method:

- Heat the nut oil in a wok over high heat.
- Add the pork mince, garlic, and ginger to the wok and cook through. Channel off any fluid to guarantee the mince is very dry.

- In a little bowl join the shellfish sauce, caster sugar, kecap manis, lime juice, and sesame oil.
- Add 66% of the sauce to the pork mince and mix through a few minutes until the sauce thickens.
- Eliminate the wok from the heat and permit the mince to cool marginally.
- In a little, dry fry container, toast the peanuts and put them to the side to cool.
- Wash, dry, and trim your lettuce leaves and spread them out on a plate.
- Split the mince combination between the lettuce cups.
- Top each San Choy Bau with salted carrot, broiled peanuts, coriander leaves, and seared shallots.
- Spoon over the leftover sauce.

36: Sheet Pan Steak

To make a sheet dish form of this exemplary meal, broil the potatoes until delicate and afterward cook everything under the oven to give it an amazing brown burn. Sheet Pan Steak and Potatoes conveys all the generous solace however practically no dishes to tidy up.

Ingredients:

- 1 head of broccoli, cut into florets
- 1/4 cup olive oil
- 2 tablespoons fresh rosemary, minced (or 2 teaspoons dry, squashed)
- 2 tablespoons balsamic vinegar
- Fit salt
- 9 cloves garlic, minced and isolated
- Fresh broke black pepper

- 1/2 pounds Yukon gold potatoes, split
- 2 pounds of level iron steak (can substitute flank steak simply try to check the inward temp)

Method:

- Preheat broiler to 450°. Line a large rimmed heating sheet with foil.
- Spot the steak in a large zipper-top pack with the 1/4 cup olive oil, 4 cloves of garlic, salt, vinegar, balsamic and pepper.
- Go to cover and let marinate at any rate 1 hour as long as 8 hours.
- Disperse potatoes and rosemary on the heating sheet and shower with 1 tablespoon of olive oil, and season with salt and pepper.
- Toss tenderly with utensils to cover and spread them out equitably.
- Cook potatoes mix until they start to brown around the edges, around 20 minutes.
- Join the leftover 2 tablespoons of olive oil, broccoli, and remaining garlic in a bowl; season with salt and pepper, and toss to cover. Spot on the heating sheet alongside the potatoes.
- Spot an ovenproof wire rack over the broccoli and potatoes. Eliminate the steak from the zip-top sack and shake off the abundance marinade. Lay the steak on the rack.
- Return the preparing sheet to the broiler and dish until a moment read thermometer embedded evenly into the focal point of meat registers 125, around 10 to 15 minutes.

- Eliminate from the broiler and let rest for 5 to 10 minutes before cutting.

37: Poached Eggs and Avocado Toasts

Make the most of your day away from work with a nutritious and healthy lunch with this Avocado Toast with Poached Egg. A basic simple avocado concoction spread on a cut of toasted wholegrain bread and finished off with a poached egg. It is flavorful. This fair may turn into a customary thing on your lunch menu.

You need a wonderfully ready avocado and a pleasant thick cut of fresh bread to toast. Since avocados become brown when the fruit is presented to the air, pound it up with a little lemon squeeze then sprinkle some salt in to draw out the flavor.

Ingredients:

- 2 eggs
- salt and pepper for ingredient
- 2 cups of wholegrain bread
- 2 tablespoons shaved Parmesan cheddar
- quartered treasure tomatoes for serving
- fresh spices (parsley, thyme, or basil) for ingredient
- 1/3 avocado (for the most part I cut it down the middle yet don't utilize every last bit of it. alright fine perhaps I do.)

Method:

- Carry a pot of water to heat (utilize sufficient water to cover the eggs when they lay in the base).

- Drop the metal edges (external edge just) of two artisan container covers into the pot so they are laying level on the base.
- When the water is bubbling, turn off the heat and cautiously break the eggs simply into each edge.
- Cover the pot and poach for 5 minutes (4 for too delicate, 4:30 for delicate, at least 5 for semi-delicate yolks).
- While the eggs are cooking, toast the bread and crush the avocado on each piece of toast.
- When the eggs are done, utilize a spatula to lift the eggs out of the water. Delicately remove the edge from the eggs (I do this privilege on the spatula, over the water) and spot the poached eggs on top of the toast.
- Sprinkle with Parmesan cheddar, salt, pepper, and fresh spices; present with the fresh quartered legacy tomatoes.

Chapter: 3 Salad & Soups

38: Veggie-Packed Cheesy Chicken Salad

These veggie-pressed dinners will have you covered from breakfast to dinner. Furthermore, these plans have close to 15 grams of sugars for every serving. Plans like Green Shakshuka and Buffalo Chicken Cauliflower Pizza are vivid, scrumptious, and brimming with supplements and nutrients.

Ingredients:

- 1 lb. uncooked slight cut chicken breasts
- 7 tablespoons diminished fat balsamic vinaigrette dressing
- 1 medium zucchini (8 oz.), cut the long way down the middle
- 1 medium red onion, cut into 1/4-inch cuts
- 4 plum (Roma) tomatoes, cut down the middle
- 6 cups torn arugula
- ½ cup disintegrated feta cheddar (2 oz.)

Method:

- Heat gas or charcoal barbecue. Brush chicken with 1 tablespoon of the dressing. Cautiously brush oil on the barbecue rack.
- Spot chicken, zucchini, and onion on flame broil over medium heat.
- Cover flame broil; cook 8 to 10 minutes, turning once, until chicken is not, at this point pink in focus and vegetables are delicate.

- Add tomato parts to flame broil throughout the previous 4 minutes of cooking.
- Reduce chicken and vegetables from flame broil to cutting board.
- Cut chicken across into slender cuts; coarsely cleave vegetables.
- In a large bowl, throw chicken, vegetables, and the leftover 6 tablespoons of dressing.
- Add arugula and cheddar; throw tenderly. Serve right away.

39: Cobb Salad with Brown Derby Dressing

The recipe contained in this Cobb Salad with French Dressing was given to me by Walt Disney World Guest Services or a Disney Chef at the eatery. The recipe in Cobb Salad with French Dressing may have been downsized by the Disney Chefs for the home culinary specialist. We love this salad. It's expensive even by Disney principles yet it genuinely is scrumptious.

Salad ingredients:

- 1/2 package watercress
- 3 eggs, hard-cooked
- 1/2 head icy mass lettuce
- 1 little pack chicory
- 2 medium tomatoes, whitened and stripped
- 1/2 head romaine lettuce
- 1/2 cups cooked turkey breast, cubed
- 2 tablespoons slashed chives
- 6 strips fresh bacon, disintegrated
- 1/2 cup blue cheddar, disintegrated

French Dressing Ingredients:

- 1/2 teaspoon sugar
- 1/2 cup water
- 1/4 tablespoons salt
- 1 clove garlic, chopped
- 1/2 cups salad oil
- 1/2 cup red wine vinegar
- 1/2 teaspoons Worcestershire sauce
- Juice of 1/2 lemon
- 1/2 teaspoon English mustard
- 1/2 cup olive oil
- 1/2 tablespoon ground dark pepper

Method for Cobb Salad:

- Slash all greens fine and mastermind in a salad bowl.
- Cut tomatoes down the middle, reduce seeds, and dice fine.
- Likewise dice the turkey, avocado, and eggs.
- Mastermind the above ingredients, just as the blue cheddar and bacon disintegrate, in straight lines across the greens.
- Mastermind the chives slantingly across the above lines.
- Present the salad at the table, then throw it with the dressing.
- Spot on chilled plates with a watercress enhancement.

Method for Dressing:

- Mix all ingredients aside from oils.
- Then add olive oil and salad oils and blend well.

- Mix well again before blending in with the salad.

40: Speedy Thai Noodle Salad

Thai Noodle Salad with the BEST EVER Peanut Sauce-stacked up with sound veggies! This veggie lover salad is incredible for potlucks and Sunday dinner - prep and keeps going as long as 5 days in the refrigerator. Gluten-free versatile. Incorporates a 35-second video.

Ingredients:

- 4 cups blend of cabbage, carrots, and radish, destroyed or ground
- 6-ounce dry noodles (earthy colored rice noodles, cushion Thai style rice noodles, soba noodles, linguini)
- 3 scallions, cut
- 1 red chime pepper, finely cut
- ½ pack cilantro, chopped (or sub basil and mint)
- ¼–½ cup broiled, squashed peanuts (embellish)
- 1 tablespoon jalapeño (finely chopped)

Method:

- Cook pasta as per bearings on the package.
- Channel and chill under cool running water.
- Throw: Place destroyed veggies, chime pepper, scallions, cilantro, and jalapeño into a serving bowl. Throw.
- Add the chilly noodles to the serving bowl and throw once more. Pour the nut sauce up and over and throw well to join.

- (However you would prefer), add stew drops if you need and serve, decorating with broiled peanuts and cilantro and a lime wedge.

41: Warm Roasted Vegetable Farro Salad

If you're in the disposition for a dinner salad that is generous, solid, and heavenly, then look no farther than this Roasted Vegetable and Farro Salad. This salad joins nutty, chewy faro with an assortment of broiled vegetables, all threw in a balsamic vinaigrette and present with disintegrated feta.

Ingredients:

- ⅔ cup broccoli florets
- 1½ cups cooked farro
- ¼ cup grape tomatoes divided
- ½ of ringer pepper, chopped
- ¼ of zucchini, cubed
- 1 tsp olive oil
- 1 tsp ocean salt + more to taste
- 1 clove garlic, shredded
- 1 tsp dried or fresh rosemary
- 4-5 kalamata olives, cut
- 2 tbsp. disintegrated goat cheddar
- ¼ cup pecan parts, slashed

Method:

- Preheat the broiler to 400°F and fix a skillet with material paper.
- Throw broccoli, tomatoes, zucchini, and ringer pepper with olive oil, rosemary, salt, and shredded garlic in a bowl until equally covered.

- Spread on arranged dish and meal in preheated broiler for 25 minutes.
- Joined broiled vegetables with cooked farro, cut olives, and pecans.
- Add salt to taste.
- Top with disintegrated goat cheddar and serve.

42: Cajun Potato, Shrimp, and Avocado Salad

We have another best recipe in our book that is Cajun Potato, Shrimp, and Avocado Salad. It is the best discontinuous fasting recipe to attempt. Many people like it and it is not difficult to make.

Ingredients:

- 2 spring onions (finely cut)
- 2 teaspoons Cajun preparing
- 1 garlic clove (shredded)
- 1 tablespoon oil (olive oil)
- 1 avocado (stripped, stoned, and cubed)
- 1 cup horse feed sprout
- Salt (to bubble potatoes)
- 300-gram potatoes (fresh potatoes, little child or talks 10 oz. divided)
- 250-gram crude shrimp (ruler prawns, 8 oz., cooked and stripped)

Method:

- Cook the potatoes in an enormous pot of delicately salted bubbling water for 10 to 15 minutes or until delicate, channel well.
- Heat the oil in a wok or large nonstick griddle/skillet.

- Add the prawns, garlic, spring onions, and Cajun preparing and pan sear for 2 to 3 minutes or until the prawns are hot.
- Mix in the potatoes and cook briefly.
- Move to serve dishes and top with the avocado and the hay fledglings and serve.

43: Simple Black Bean Soup

It is a basic and solid soup made with canned dark beans and regular ingredients! This delightful dark bean soup is veggie-lover, without gluten, and vegan. This soup is ideal for lunch, occupied weeknights, or taking care of an eager group. Our whole family cherishes this soup and we as a whole get energized when it's on the menu! It hits the recognize without fail.

Ingredients:

- 1 medium red onion, finely chopped
- 2 tbsp. extra-virgin olive oil
- 2 cloves garlic, shredded
- 1 tbsp. tomato glue
- 1 tbsp. shredded jalapeños
- salt
- 1 tsp. bean stew powder
- Freshly ground dark pepper
- 1/2 tsp. cumin
- 3 (15-oz.) jars dark beans, with fluid
- 1 bay leaf
- 1 qt. low-sodium chicken or vegetable stock
- acrid cream, for embellish
- Cleaved fresh cilantro, for embellish

- Cut avocado, to decorate

Method:

- In an enormous pot over medium heat, heat oil. Add onion and cook until delicate and clear, around 5 minutes.
- Add jalapeños and garlic and cook until fragrant, around 2 minutes.
- Add tomato glue, mix to cover vegetables, and cook about a brief more. Season with salt, bean stew powder, pepper, and cumin and mix to cover.
- Add dark beans with their fluid and chicken stock. Mix soup, add cove leaf and heat to the point of boiling.
- Quickly decrease to a stew and let stew until marginally diminished around 15 minutes. Reduce inlet leaf.
- Utilizing a drenching blender or food processor, mix the soup to wanted consistency.
- Present with a touch of sharp cream, cut avocado, and cilantro.

Chapter: 4 Dinner

This Chicken Fried Cauliflower Rice is not difficult to make and can be filled in as your principal dish or as a side dish. It's low in focuses, low in carbs, and loaded up with veggies and protein. It is a fast and simple Asian one container supper recipe that the whole family will cherish.

Ingredients:

- 2 big eggs
- 1 tablespoon sesame oil
- 1/2 cup chopped onion
- 2 tablespoons olive or avocado oil
- 1 clove garlic, crushed
- 1 teaspoon fresh ginger, crushed
- 4 teaspoons soy sauce, separated
- 1 cup cooked chicken
- 1 pound riced cauliflower
- 1/2 cup chopped scallions
- 1 tablespoon stew glue

Method:

- Heat oil in a big oven or wok over medium heat.
- Add the onion and cook, mixing regularly, until clear.
- Add the ginger, garlic, and chicken to the container and keep cooking for 2 minutes.

- Add the cauliflower to the oven and sprinkle with 3 teaspoons (1 tablespoon) of soy sauce and stew glue.
- Mix well and cook for 3 minutes or until the cauliflower has mollified.
- Push the cauliflower rice to the side of the dish and break the eggs into the unfilled space in the container. Sprinkle with 1 teaspoon soy sauce and scramble.
- When eggs are cooked through, mix the eggs into the rice.
- Remove from the heat and stir in the scallions.
- Sprinkle with sesame oil and serve.

45: Wild Cajun Spiced Salmon

Cajun Salmon with a simple natively constructed preparation made with flavors you as of now have in your washroom that can be heated, cooked, dish singed, or barbecued. This solid supper is prepared in under fifteen minutes and comparable to any eatery variant.

Cajun Salmon that is hot, smoky, and prepared right away makes for a simple and solid supper that can be cooked inside or outside on the flame broil. Serve it warm or cold for a protein-stuffed supper that is scrumptious. We likewise make this Blackened Salmon and Brown Sugar Salmon consistently, so add these to your go-to salmon plans.

Ingredients:

- 3 tsp olive oil, separated
- 2 6 oz. filets of salmon
- 2 tbsp. Cajun preparing
- Legitimate salt + broke black pepper, to taste

Method:

- Preheat the stove to 425 degrees C.
- Brush a preparing dish or oven with 1 tsp olive oil.
- Put salmon filets down into dish — skin-side down if they have skin.
- Brush 1 tsp of olive oil over each filet.
- Sprinkle with Kosher salt + broke black pepper.
- Sprinkle each filet with 1 tbsp. of Cajun preparing each, tapping and kneading the flavoring into the filet like a rub.
- Rub onto the sides of the filets too.
- Spot in the broiler and heat for 15 minutes or until filets effectively drop.
- The safe inward temperature for fish is 62.8 °C/145 °F.

46: Healthy Beef Stroganoff

This Healthy Beef Stroganoff recipe is outstanding both for what it offers—all the smooth, comfortable kind of the exemplary recipe, eased up with a couple of solid ingredient trades and made simpler in the simmering pot—just as for what it doesn't. This stewing pot meat stroganoff is made without canned soup.

Ingredients:

- 1 tablespoon margarine
- ½ teaspoon salt
- 1 teaspoon arranged mustard
- 2-pound meat hurl cook
- ½ teaspoon ground black pepper
- salt and ground black pepper to taste

- ⅓ cup white wine
- ¼ cup generally useful flour
- ½ pound white mushrooms, cut
- 1 ¼ cups decreased sodium meat stock, separated
- ⅓ cup light acrid cream
- 4 green onions, cut (white and green parts)
- 2 tablespoons spread, partitioned

Method:

- Remove any fat and cartilage from the meal and cut into strips 1/2-inch thick by 2-inches in length.
- Sprinkle with 1/2 teaspoon salt and 1/2 teaspoon pepper.
- Soften 1 tablespoon margarine in a large oven over medium heat.
- Add mushrooms and green onions and cook, mixing once in a while, until mushrooms are sautéed, around 6 minutes.
- Remove to a bowl and add 1 tablespoon margarine to the oven.
- Cook and mix one a large portion of the hamburger strips until caramelized, around 5 minutes, then remove to a bowl.
- Rehash with the excess spread and hamburger strips.
- Empty wine into the hot oven and deglaze the container, scraping up any sautéed bits.
- Join flour and 1/4 cup meat stock in a container with a firmly fitting cover and shake until consolidated.
- Stir into the oven, racing until smooth.

- Stir in the excess stock and mustard, then return the meat to the container.
- Bring to a stew. Cover and stew until the meat are delicate, around 60 minutes.
- Stir in the readied mushrooms and the acrid cream five minutes before serving. Heat momentarily and sprinkle with salt and pepper.

47: Better Potato Nachos

This tasty and solid yam nachos recipe contains 47.9 grams of protein and 6.4 grams of fiber in only one serving. These yam nachos are solid, clean, and effectively made paleo and vegetarian, as well. Solid Potato Nachos is a sound option in contrast to customary nachos. This recipe is not difficult to follow and is kid-accommodating as well. All you need is a yam, black beans, chicken, and conventional nacho ingredients to make this fast, simple, fun recipe that is diabetes agreeable, gluten-free, heart-healthy, and low in sodium.

Ingredients:

- 18oz lean meat mince
- 14oz can Mexican-style tomatoes
- 23oz potatoes, daintily cut
- 1 onion, finely cleaved
- 15oz can gentle stew beans
- olive shower oil
- ½ cup ground fat-free cheddar
- To serve
- 2 spring onions, finely slashed
- ⅓ cup fat-free harsh cream
- slashed fresh coriander

Method:

- Preheat broiler to 375°F. Cook potatoes in bubbling water for 8-10 minutes until somewhat delicate.
- 2Brown mince in a non-stick oven. Add onion. Cook for a couple of moments.
- Add beans and tomatoes.
- Cook for 4-5 minutes.
- Mastermind a large portion of the potatoes in a big ovenproof dish or split between 4 person dishes.
- Shower with a little olive oil.
- Spoon over mince. Orchestrate remaining potatoes up and over.
- Splash with oil. Sprinkle with cheddar.
- Prepare for 25 minutes.
- Present with acrid cream, spring onions, and coriander.

48: Sheet Pan Chicken and Brussel Sprouts

This is a real stove-to-table sheet-container supper brimming with delicate, crunchy Brussels sprouts and firm, lemony chicken. A simple lemon-and-spice compound spread sprinkles both the chicken and fledglings, which are then finished off with slender lemon cuts that become crunchy in the broiler, offering a decent textural component and a splendid sprinkle of shading and flavor. The key is to cut the lemon adjusts nearly paper-flimsy, so they can fresh up and lose their harshness.

Ingredients:

- 4 cups Brussels sprouts, quartered
- ¾ teaspoon salt, separated
- ½ teaspoon ground cumin
- ¾ teaspoon ground pepper, separated
- ½ teaspoon dried thyme
- ½ teaspoon dried thyme
- 2 tablespoons extra-virgin olive oil, separated
- 1 pound yams, cut into 1/2-inch wedges
- 1 ¼ pound boneless, skinless chicken thighs, managed

Method:

- Preheat broiler to 425 degrees F.
- Toss yams with 1 tablespoon oil and 1/4 teaspoon each salt and pepper in a large bowl.
- Spread equitably on a rimmed preparing sheet. Broil for 15 minutes.
- Toss Brussels sprouts with the leftover 1 tablespoon oil and 1/4 teaspoon each salt and pepper in the bowl.
- Stir into the yams on the preparing sheet.
- Sprinkle chicken with cumin, thyme, and the leftover 1/4 teaspoon of each salt and pepper. Spot on top of the vegetables.
- Broil until the chicken is cooked through and the vegetables are delicate, 10 to 15 minutes more.
- Move the chicken to a serving platter. Mix vinegar into the vegetables and present with the chicken.

This salad may help you to remember a cocktail or a wedge salad. Consider well drink trims, like celery, parsley, green olives, anchovies, or bacon, when choosing what else to add to this dish.

Ingredients:

- 2 tbsp. red wine vinegar
- 2 tbsp. olive oil
- 2 tsp. Worcestershire sauce
- 1/2 tsp. Tabasco
- 2 tsp. arranged horseradish pressed dry
- 1/2 tsp. celery seeds
- Kosher salt and pepper
- 2 celery stems, daintily cut
- 1-16-ounce cherry tomatoes, split
- 1/2 little red onion, daintily cut
- 1 little head green-leaf lettuce, leaves torn
- 1/4 c. level leaf parsley, finely cleaved
- 4 little bone-in pork slashes (1 in. thick, about 2¼ lbs. all-out)

Method:

- Heat barbecue to medium-high.
- In a big bowl, whisk together oil, vinegar, Worcestershire sauce, horseradish, Tabasco, celery seeds, and ¼ teaspoon salt. Toss with tomatoes, celery, and onion.

- Sprinkle pork slashes with 1/2 teaspoon each salt and pepper and barbecue until brilliant earthy colored and just cooked through, 5 to 7 minutes for every side.
- Overlay parsley into tomatoes and serve over pork and greens.

50: Slow-Cooker Black Eyed Peas

This Slow Cooked Black Eyed Peas recipe requires only a couple of minutes of prep, then everything gets toss in the sluggish cooker! Black peered toward peas are the ideal solace food. Made with an extra ham bone and stewed in a rich delectable stock, these Slow Cooker Black Eyed Peas and Collard Greens are a tasty expansion to your Fresh Year's Day menu.

Ingredients:

- salt, to taste
- 1 shape chicken bouillon
- 6 cups water
- 1 onion, chopped
- 2 cloves garlic, chopped
- 1 pound dried black peered toward peas, arranged and flushed
- 1 jalapeno Chile, cultivated and crushed
- 1 red ringer pepper, stemmed, cultivated, and chopped
- 1 teaspoon ground black pepper
- 8 ounces chopped ham
- 4 cuts bacon, cleaved
- ½ teaspoon cayenne pepper
- 1 ½ teaspoons cumin

Method:

- Empty the water into a lethargic cooker, add the bouillon block, and mix to break down.
- Join the black peered toward peas, onion, salt, Chile pepper, garlic, jalapeno pepper, bacon, cayenne pepper, ham, cumin, and pepper; mix to mix.
- Cover the lethargic cooker and cook on Low for 6 to 8 hours until the beans are delicate.

51: Salmon and Veggies at 5:30 P.M.

Barbecued salmon and veggies make for a beautiful and adjusted fish supper that is prepared in only minutes. The flame broil turns the salmon flaky and sodden while softening the fresh pepper and onion pieces. Balance the supper with earthy-colored rice or quinoa. This carb-cognizant dinner is loaded with protein and nutrients. Transform it into a sheet oven supper recipe if you don't have a meal dish.

Ingredients:

- salt, to taste
- pepper, to taste
- 4 cloves garlic, crushed
- 2 teaspoons ginger
- 4 tablespoons olive oil
- 4 tablespoons lemon juice
- 2 tablespoons fresh thyme
- 2 salmon filets
- 2 lb. little red potato (910 g), or yellow, quartered
- 1 package asparagus, about 1 pound (455g)

Method:

- Preheat the stove to 400°F (200°C).
- Cover a sheet dish with foil or material paper. Spread out potatoes in the oven and sprinkle with olive oil. Sprinkle with salt, pepper, 2 cloves of garlic, and 1 tablespoon lemon juice.
- Heat for 30 minutes.
- Make salmon coating.
- Join salt, pepper, 2 garlic cloves, 1 tablespoon thyme, ginger, 2 tablespoons of olive oil, and 2 tablespoons of lemon juice. Blend well.
- Remove potatoes from the broiler and push them to the top or side of your oven.
- Spot your salmon filets on the container.
- Brush the two sides of the salmon with the coating.
- Spot asparagus on the dish and top with 1 tablespoon olive oil, salt, 1 tablespoon lemon squeeze, and pepper.
- Sprinkle 1 tsp of thyme on the potatoes and asparagus.
- Prepare for 10-12 minutes. (The salmon should piece effectively with a fork when it's prepared.) Enjoy!

52: Poached Egg with Asparagus and Tomato

This supper is a fast and simple path for any recipe phobe to prepare an overly scrumptious dish in a matter of moments. With their various medical advantages, eggs are extraordinary at any time and taste scrumptious when presented with fresh asparagus lances.

Ingredients:

- 1 tablespoon honey
- 1 tablespoon Dijon mustard
- 2 shallots, shaved slight
- ½ cup olive oil
- 1 lemon, supreme, and juiced*
- Coarse salt and fresh broke pepper, to taste
- 2 garlic cloves, crushed
- 2 packages asparagus, bottoms managed
- 4 Creole tomatoes, cut in thick adjusts
- 6 tablespoons parmesan, ground
- 4 eggs

Method:

- Carry a big pot of salted water to stew and keep prepared.
- In the mixing bowl, add Dijon mustard, shallots, honey, lemon Supremes, and juice. Race in olive oil and sprinkle with salt and pepper. Put dressing in a safe spot.
- In the large oven, add a sprinkle of olive oil and singe asparagus stems in clumps with a spot of crushed garlic. Sprinkle with salt and pepper.
- Spot stems in a single layer in the oven so they don't steam and overcook.
- If planning early, place promptly into the cooler, serve chilled.
- Have everything plated and all set before poaching eggs, as they are time-touchy.
- On large plates mastermind cuts of tomato, marginally covering one another.

- Shower tomatoes with olive oil and sprinkle with salt and pepper.
- Gap and organize singed asparagus on plates.
- To poach eggs, add a sprinkle of white vinegar to a pot of stewing water.
- Whirl spoon around in your water to make it move in roundabout movement and afterward break and drop your eggs into the center.
- Delicately twirl water.
- Poach 2-4 minutes to cook, or until whites are firm to contact and focus are giggly.

To gather, place one poached egg on top of each heap of asparagus. 53: Yogurt with Blueberries

A simple blend of Greek yogurt and blueberries gets an additional dash of pleasantness from brilliant honey. It's the ideal equilibrium of protein and fiber to keep you empowered. These two food varieties draw out the best in one another.

The high fiber substance of the berries (just about four grams for every cup) reinforces the sound microbes found in yogurt, also known as probiotics, assisting it with enduring the dangerous excursion through the stomach-related lot. Once in the gut, the probiotics assist the body with engrossing the solvent fiber of the blueberries.

Ingredients:

- ¼ cup blueberries
-
- Blend vinaigrette and delicately spoon over the egg, asparagus, and tomatoes.
- Get done with freshly ground parmesan and serve right away.
- 1 cup nonfat plain Greek yogurt

Method:

- Spot yogurt in a bowl and top with blueberries.

Add the Mediterranean contort to your plate with this Feta and Tomato Omelets recipe with feta cheddar, black olives, and tomato. Greek omelet is an exceptionally flexible dish one can appreciate at any time. It very well may be filled in as a filling high-energy breakfast, a quick bite with some dry town bread, or even dinner.

This Feta and Tomato Omelets recipe is truly simple to plan and incorporates basic ingredients, however, the taste is truly flawless and fresh. You will adore the blend of feta and tomato.

Ingredients:

- 3 black Kalamata olives
- 1/2 tomato, slashed into shapes
- 60g/2 oz. feta cheddar disintegrated
- 2 tbsps. olive oil
- a squeeze dried oregano
- 3 large eggs
- ground Graviera cheddar to decorate
- salt and freshly ground pepper

Method:

- To make this heavenly Greek omelet recipe start by setting up the ingredients first.
- Remove the seeds and add juice from the tomato and cut the tissue into little 3D squares. Put in a safe spot.

- Remove the pits from the olives and cut them into little pieces. Put in a safe spot.
- Disintegrate the feta cheddar with your hands or utilizing a fork and set it aside.
- Break the eggs in a bowl and sprinkle with salt and pepper. Beat the eggs with a fork until consolidated.
- Heat a little medium nonstick griddle over medium heat.
- Add 2 tbsps. olive oil and the beaten eggs. Utilizing a spatula, drag the omelet towards the one finish of the oven and slant the dish to allow the crude eggs to fill the unfilled side.
- Rehash this interaction for approx. 1-2 minutes until the omelet is cooked. (the eggs are set yet the top is still marginally clammy)
- Remove the dish from the heat and add the tomato, feta cheddar, olives, oregano.
- Slip the spatula under the omelet, tip to release, and delicately overlay the omelet fifty-fifty.
- Sprinkle with ground cheddar and serve.

55: Spicy Chocolate Keto Fat Bombs

Keto chocolate is high in fat and sugar-free for a low carb contort, however all you'll taste is smooth, velvety dull chocolate flavor combined with an impactful zest blend that makes certain to warm you up a bit! It's so natural to make chocolate at home with only a couple of ingredients.

Try it and see with your own eyes. These scrumptious and delish keto fat bombs make certain to be hit. Fill in as keto pastries, keto snacks, keto sweet treat, or make to take to parties. These are even raved about by people who don't follow a ketogenic diet/lifestyle.

You can add a wide range of additional ingredients to the focal point of the hot cocoa bombs, sprinkles to the outside, or considerably more dissolved chocolate. They look so extravagant and beautiful, so normally, they are stunning endowments as well.

Ingredients:

- ⅓ cup cocoa powder
- ½ cup sugar
- ⅓ cup weighty cream powder
- 7 oz. ChocZero sugar free chocolate chips (1 sack of milk or dim chips)

Optional:

- sugar free sprinkles
- 1 tsp coconut oil
- ¼ cup ChocZero without sugar white chocolate chips

Method:

- Microwave the sugar free chocolate chips for 30 seconds.
- Mix. If they aren't softened microwave at 15 seconds spans, mixing after each.
- When they are about 75% softened simply mix until they are liquefied.
- Spoon a stacking teaspoon into every cavity of a 2-inch circle form. Utilize the rear of the teaspoon to push the chocolate up the edges.

- As it sets keep pushing chocolate up the sides to make a thicker shell.
- Spot a storing tablespoon of the hot cocoa blend inside a large portion of the circles.
- Spoon on dissolved chocolate around the edge.
- Top with the second 50% of the circle.
- Optional: Drizzle with extra liquefied chocolate blended in with 1 teaspoon of coconut oil and top with sprinkles.
- Refrigerate until fixed.
- Spot a hot cocoa bomb into a mug.
- Pour 6-ounce of hot milk on chocolate bomb.
- Mix until smooth.

Conclusion:

Thus, in conclusion, just by following a two times per week 24-hour Intermittent fasting plan for half a month you will get a healthy and slim body. However, if you can improve your diet when that you don't fast then you will lose more weight, and assuming you can adhere to this system, you will keep the load off without falling back on any accident diets or diets that are only difficult to adhere to.

Intermittent fasting has been appeared to reduce the kind of white platelet called monocytes. Monocytes are connected with body irritation. By reducing inflammation, constant musculoskeletal agonies can be improved. Cancer cells ordinarily feed on glucose. Blood glucose is high when we nibble and eat much of the time. Alternately, when we fast Intermittently, we burn fat.

Since most cancer cells can't benefit from fat disease hazard exercises. A few studies show that Intermittent fasting helps the body with clearing out toxins and harmed cells. This purifying and refinement lessens sleepiness and languor and helps support energy.

When starting with Intermittent fasting, make sure you start simple, getting your body used to avoiding a day once per week, then maybe two. Also, go slowly when working out during this changing time, until you begin to feel like you're ready to take a full burden in your exercise program. This will not take long, and indeed, will leave you wanting more.

If you're looking for a way to speed up your fat loss and continue to work out, then you need to investigate Intermittent fasting. You might be satisfied with exactly how compelling it tends to be at easily lessening your caloric intake while letting your adequate energy finish your exercises.

For somebody who is sound and needs to attempt Intermittent fasting, it should not be troublesome. Nonetheless, people with dietary problems, diabetes, diseases, people who are finished or underweight should counsel certified health proficient before beginning with this kind of eating pattern.

To conclude, we need to comprehend that Intermittent fasting is not a magic pill. A certified nutritionist can fabricate a successful weight management program with Intermittent fasting by consolidating a sound diet of nutritious genuine food sources with customary exercise and satisfactory rest.

Mediterranean Diet Recipes

The Complete Cookbook for Long Lasting Weight Loss and Healthy Lifstyle

By Sarah Clark

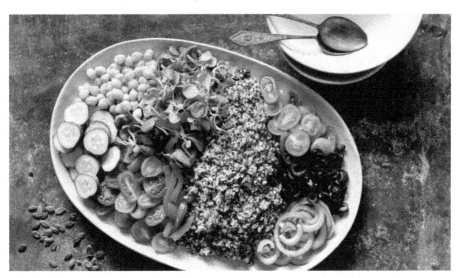

INTRODUCTION

The Mediterranean diet is becoming more popular because it is not based on propagated trends. Rather, it is a model which comes from many years of use. This diet is encouraged by many traditional eating trends of the Mediterranean era. The Mediterranean diet consists of healthy and fresh plant food like vegetables, fish, fruits, whole grains, legumes, nuts, seafood, and olives. They combine this with red meat and dairy products. It is because red meat is an uncommon source of protein in the Mediterranean Diet.

The Mediterranean diet is very healthy because all the foods are less processed. Cooking or processing food deprives it of healthy nutrients. However, in the Mediterranean diet, lightly cooked foods are eaten. Some foods are eaten raw. If red meat is served, it is also clipped with extra fat.

So, we accept that following the Mediterranean diet has various health benefits. This diet provides rich fiber, vitamins, healthy fats, minerals, protein, and many other essential fatty acids essential for the body to keep healthy and prevent diseases like cancer and heart disease. This diet has been found to cure many other diseases like high blood pressure, type II diabetes, angina, and arthritis.

So, hopefully, you are convinced to follow the diet Mediterranean. Now, you'd want to figure out how to prepare Mediterranean diet recipes. For your help, we are publishing an excellent cookbook in the market, Mediterranean Diet Recipes. It is a great publication dedicated to people who follow this diet. The book will help you live a healthy and long life.

All of these Mediterranean diet recipes are suitable for you. These recipes have been included as a healthy supplement. So, it's your time to try these delicious, healthy Mediterranean diet recipes!

Mushroom, Spinach, Tomato Frittata with Feta Cheese

Many Mediterranean food recipes include a lot of fresh and colorful vegetables. These are useful for a healthy life. Try to replace your favorite herbs and vegetable with a personalized and unique Mediterranean meal.

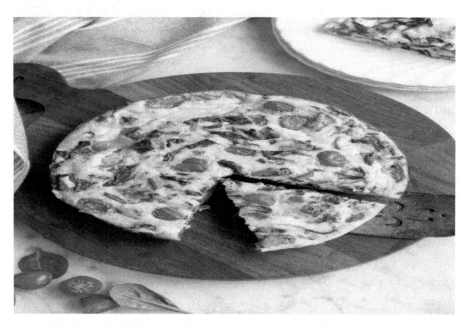

Ingredients:

- 6 eggs
- 1 onion (chopped)
- 2 tomatoes (sliced)
- 1/4 tsp pepper
- 1 garlic clove (minced)
- 1/4 tsp salt
- 8 oz, or 3 cups mushrooms (sliced)
- 1 Tabspn extra virgin olive oil
- 10 oz, or 1 bag fresh spinach (chopped)
- 1/2 tsp oregano (OR any your favorite herb)

- 1/4 cup milk (reduced fat or skim)
- 1/2 cup feta cheese (smashed)

Method:

- ✓ Add oil to the non-stick ovenproof pan.
- ✓ Over medium heat, cook onion, pepper, mushrooms, salt, garlic, and herbs.
- ✓ Stir for approximately 8 minutes to prevent sticking. Stir until all fluid is removed.
- ✓ Now add spinach. Cover it. Cook it for at least 5 minutes when the spinach is just wilting.
- ✓ Beat eggs in a mixing bowl.
- ✓ Add eggs and cheese to the pan comprising cooked vegetables. Stir gently to mix them and turn heat to low.
- ✓ Place all the sliced tomatoes on top and cook them uncovered at least for about 10 minutes. Cook them until a slight amount of juice leftovers.
- ✓ Now place under the grill for 3 to 5 minutes till set.
- ✓ Slice it and serve with salad or fresh serveal vegetables sprinkled with some virgin olive oil.

Recipe: 2

Grilled Shrimp Salad

The grilled Shrimp Salad recipe is the perfect option for your summer dinner desires. The recipe is healthy and full of Grilled Shrimp flavor. This a delicious recipe that makes your dinner perfect during the warm months of summer. I love this recipe as it is healthy and easy to make.

Ingredients:

- One Avocado
- 10 - 12 large shrimp
- One bunch of asparagus
- A Cup full of extra virgin olive oil
- One cup of lime juice
- Two teaspoons of garlic (powdered)
- Two to three zucchini (as per your requirements0
- Two cups of freshly basil leave (sliced)
- A mug full of red mauve tart (preferably a tart that has a sour taste)
- One spoon of mustard (must have a thick yellow paste having a spiky flavor)
- Two cups of salad kinds including radicchio, endive, and butter lettuce

Method:

- ✓ Make a mixture of lime juice, olive oil, chopped fresh garlic, pesto, and red vinegar.
- ✓ Now reserve the shrimp in 1 ½ of the salad dressing (for half an hour).
- ✓ Place the shrimp on the bayonet.
- ✓ Chop asparagus and zucchini sideways.
- ✓ Lay the zucchini, shrimp, and asparagus onto the oven grill.
- ✓ Heat it until prepared.

- ✓ Now place all of the heated things in a basin.
- ✓ In the end, cut up avocado and put it to the heated stuff.

Roasted Mediterranean Style Leg of Lamb with Artichokes

Here is another best Mediterranean diet recipe for you. This recipe is featuring such traditional Mediterranean foods as garlic, lamb, and artichokes. The recipe is healthy and has a good flavor.

Ingredients:

- 2 tsp salt
- 4lb leg of lamb
- 1 tsp pepper
- 1 cup, OR 250 ml water
- 1 garlic clove (minced)
- 1 tsp oregano (chopped finely)
- 8 oz, OR 1 cup of tomato passata
- 9 oz artichoke hearts (marinated, tinned, or frozen)

Method:

- ✓ Heat oven to 325º F.
- ✓ Scrub the combined salt, pepper, and oregano into the lamb.
- ✓ Place lamb on the stand in a shallow baking pan.
- ✓ Bake it in the oven for almost 2 1/2 hours.
- ✓ Now, it's time to remove the lamb and baking stand from the oven.
- ✓ Ditch fat from baking juices. Place lamb back in a pan (place it without the baking rack)
- ✓ Combine passata, garlic, and water, and pour over lamb.
- ✓ Place the sliced lemon on the top of the lamb.
- ✓ Now place artichokes around lamb in baking dish.

- ✓ Bake for more than 30-60 minutes (basting with sauce until meat thermometer reaches 175-180º F.)
- ✓ Now serve it with salad. You can also serve it with roast vegetables such as pumpkin, potatoes, and sweet potato.

White Bean Dip

White Bean Dip is a healthy, quick, and easy recipe that requires only a few ingredients and just five minutes to be ready. The recipe is thick and creamy. With three different distinctions comprised in the recipe, there is something for everybody at your game day party or holiday.

Ingredients:

- One small onion (chopped)
- One crimson pepper
- One large spoon of powdered garlic
- Two containers of blue beans or flotilla
- Extra olive oil

Method:

- ✓ Fry the chopped onion in olive oil.
- ✓ Add a large spoon of squashed garlic and slashed raw red pepper in olive oil till it gets hot and the color of the onion gets clear.
- ✓ Draw off all the water that remains and wash 2 tins of gray-blue beans.
- ✓ Place all constituents in a food grater and mix till it gets delicate and soft.
- ✓ Blend it with marine salt and pepper for flavor and on top of it sprinkle with olive oil and serve up with hot portions of wheat bread.

Recipe: 5

Healthy Greek Salad

There are many ways to make the salad because it comprises your preferable ingredients, and contains sufficient flavor, and keeps your advantage so you keep on coming back more. This Healthy Greek Salad recipe is our interpretation of an exemplary top choice. Its remarkable mix of flavors makes sure to make it a diet staple in your home. This recipe takes the whole of the best components of the Mediterranean diet and utilizes them to catch the embodiment of the flavor of the region many of us are so enchanted with.

Ingredients:

- 1 Spanish onion
- 3 tomatoes (chopped)
- 4 teaspoons fresh lemon juice
- 1 1/2 teaspoon oregano
- 8 pitted Kalamata olives (chopped)
- 1/4 cup extra virgin olive oil
- 1 cup feta cheese (reduced fat)
- Salt and pepper (as desired)
- 2 cucumbers (chopped, peeled, or sliced)

Method:

- ✓ Combine oregano, lemon juice, pepper, and salt olive oil.
- ✓ Combine tomatoes, cucumbers, and onion in a suitably sized salad bowl.
- ✓ Sprinkle over salad.
- ✓ Place feta cheese and olives attractively on the top.

Recipe: 6

Vegetable Bean Soup

In case you're searching for more vegan soup recipes that will fill you up and give you energy, then this Mediterranean White Bean Soup is certainly one to try. It's a very simple recipe to make with no extravagant ingredients or convoluted advances. Furthermore, you can utilize canned white beans to make it considerably quicker and simpler. Vegetable bean soup at one time can be served to a limit of eight persons. This simple vegetable and bean soup meets up rapidly and makes a healthy and good supper. You can undoubtedly customize it with whatever veggies you have available.

Ingredients:

- A cup full of kidney beans
- Two averaged sized onions (chopped)
- A cup full of white bean salt
- One carrot (peeled and chopped)
- One roughly rhizome (sliced)
- One bay leaf (roughly chopped)
- One horde of dill (chopped)
- A cup of spinach leaves
- 3 cabbage leaves
- Black pepper
- 1 glass full of rice (washed rice)
- Parmesan cheese (to be used as the topping)
- Olive oil (for giving a damp feel to the dish)
- Three endive leaves

Method:

- ✓ Soak dried beans in cold water for about an hour and after that draw off the water.
- ✓ Get a big dish loaded up with saline water and warm it. Then put the beans, carrot, onions, celery, and bay leaves.
- ✓ When the water is bubbling, reduce the heat so the soup or chowder steadily stews.
- ✓ Next 45 minutes, check for the flexibility of the beans, and if they are still hardened, keep bubbling until they become soft.
- ✓ After the underlying interaction, put in cabbage, dill, and endive leaves. Add salt and pepper according to your requirements.
- ✓ Low heat up the mixture for around 30 minutes.
- ✓ Put in the rice and cook it for fifteen minutes with the cover on.
- ✓ Sprinkle olive oil and cheddar over it and it is prepared to serve.

Traditional Tabbouleh

It is healthy, reviving, and delicious. This recipe is the conventional way that they make it in Lebanon. This latest recipe beauty and flavor is in its effortlessness which is the thing that makes it so flexible. Keep the integrity of this recipe and don't add some other ingredients. Tabbouleh is a particularly extraordinary salad. It joins every one of the exemplary elements of the Mediterranean: cucumbers, tomatoes, spices, olive oil, and lemon. While it's anything but a Greek dish, it joins ingredients basic in Greek cuisine, and people love it.

Ingredients:

- Juice of 1 lemon
- 1/4 cup bulgur
- 1/2 cup boiling water
- 1 onion (finely chopped)
- 1 cup parsley (chopped)
- 5 tomatoes (chopped)
- 2 teaspoons extra virgin olive oil
- Pinch of salt (if required)
- 1/4 cup fresh mint (chopped)

Method:

- ✓ Add bubbling water to bulgur in a little bowl.
- ✓ Blend, then cover. Stand around an hour.
- ✓ Drain off any extra water.
- ✓ Consolidate remaining ingredients in a bowl.
- ✓ Add mollified bulgur and blend well.

Spaghetti with Fresh Tomato

It is important to impart this beautiful Spaghetti with Fresh Tomato Sauce. I have been getting a charge out of tomatoes for quite a long time in such countless various recipes. The success of this recipe lies in the tomatoes. Fresh tomatoes taste so great; they need little else to help their innate flavor. It can be served to four people.

Ingredients:

- Four garlic pieces
- Six hundred grams of thick tomatoes
- Oregano (Chopped)
- Three big spoons of extra virgin olive oil
- Fifty grams of piccante pecorino (finely chopped)
- Basil leaves (Thinly grated)
- Red or black spice & salt

Method:

- ✓ Boil tomatoes in water; take them out after a lot of time and afterward strip them of their skin and cut them into little pieces by hand.
- ✓ You can take out every one of the seeds cautiously however the vast majority don't. Place the ground tomatoes in a dish bowl alongside squashed garlic, olive oil, oregano, and basil leaves.
- ✓ Put the tomatoes in bubbling water; eliminate them following a couple of moments, strip, and cut them into little pieces by hand.
- ✓ Get rid of the water and the seeds. Put a fabric over a bowl for 1 hour so every one of the ingredients inside the bowl gets doused.

- ✓ After 60 minutes, bubble and cook the spaghetti, hack the pecorino, and put it in a similar bowl. On top of this, sprinkle black or red pepper according as you would prefer.
- ✓ Serve it with red wine.

Daube De Cuisse De Canard

Daubes are very popular. Lamb and beef are commonly utilized, however so are down and domestic fowl. This recipe comes from Franck Cerutti, proprietor culinary expert of Don Camillo in Nice, where true local cooking is presented in a refined however not sissified structure. To go with it, serve polenta or gnocchi tossed with Parmigiano-Reggiano and butter.

Ingredients:

- 10 duck legs
- Butter
- 2 carrots (cubed)
- 4 shallots (chopped)
- 2 stalks celery (cubed)
- 2 to 3 sprigs of fresh thyme
- 1 tablespoon flour
- Extra-virgin olive oil
- 2 to 3 sprigs of fresh rosemary
- 2 bay leaves
- 2 onions (chopped)
- Freshly ground pepper
- 2 sprigs of fresh thyme
- 6 juniper berries
- Salt
- 1 tablespoon glace de viande (optional
- 1 bottle dry red wine (750-milliliter)

Method:

- ✓ Cut duck legs in half.
- ✓ Put a lot of oil and margarine in a big weighty lined pot and cook gradually in clumps, turning habitually until delicately caramelized on all sides.
- ✓ Return all cooked duck pieces to the pot.
- ✓ Add carrots, shallots, onions, and celery.
- ✓ Increase heat and cook for 5 minutes, mixing regularly.
- ✓ Transform all ingredients out of the dish into a colander.
- ✓ Let drain 5 to 10 minutes.
- ✓ Place ingredients in an enormous terracotta or glass heating dish that can be covered.
- ✓ Sprinkle flour over ingredients and mix until it vanishes.
- ✓ Add thyme, wine, bay leaves, rosemary, and juniper berries.
- ✓ Serve to taste with salt and pepper.
- ✓ Cover firmly and prepare at 325 degrees, without lifting top, for 2 hours.
- ✓ Mix in glace de viande when daube is done
- ✓ Serve 3 pieces for every person.

Mediterranean Tomato Sauce

The well-eminent Mediterranean diet has been seen as an ideal system of a heart-friendly dietary routine by various food and wellbeing experts around the world. This view comes from the moderately low paces of heart and cardiovascular infirmities among people living in the nations and regions that border the Mediterranean Sea.

Ingredients:

- One fresh garlic (chopped)
- One (big) spoon of olive oil
- One cup of red wine
- Sprinkled marine salt and black pepper
- Two big spoons of grated basil leave
- Twelve tomatoes (peeled and slightly crushed)

Method:

- ✓ Put fresh tomatoes in a pan and boil them for longer than a minute.
- ✓ After that drain, the excess water, strip the tomatoes and cut them.
- ✓ Deep heat the olive oil in a pan and afterward drop in the onion and garlic.
- ✓ Heat them for over 3 minutes, stir them until they become flexible.
- ✓ Add a little spice, red wine, black pepper and salt, and stew.
- ✓ Cook the pasta for 15-20 minutes.
- ✓ Put the sauce in the refrigerator for three days. Mediterranean pureed tomatoes can be frozen up for a time of four to five months.

Recipe: 11

Falafel Flatbread

Falafel flatbread is a vegetarian and gluten-free bread. It is made using a mix of vegetables, spices, and chickpeas. It's an extraordinary interpretation of a conventional flatbread that is overflowing with fresh and exquisite Mediterranean flavors. Make this recipe and enjoy your day!

Ingredients:

- 1 Radish/8g Radish, Red, Unprepared, Average
- 30g Salad, Mixed Leaf, Average
- 3 Falafels/75g Falafel, Cauldron Foods
- 1 Mushroom/7g Mushrooms, Button, Raw, Average
- 1 Small Portion/14g Cucumber, Average
- 15g Carrots, Raw, Average, Grated
- 20g Houmous, Reduced Fat, Average
- 1 Flatbread/33g Bread, Folded, Flatbread, Plain, Sainsbury's

Method:

- ✓ Spread a flatbread, or pitta, with houmous, top with blended leaves, warmed falafel, grated carrot, mushroom, radish, and cucumber.
- ✓ Cut the mushroom, radish, and dice the cucumber. Mesh the carrot and heat the falafel if you like.

Chicken with Tomato-Balsamic Pan Sauce

Brisk sautéing a chicken breast and making a pan sauce is a simple method to put dinner on the table on any bustling weeknight. Sweet and acidic tomatoes and balsamic vinegar mix so well together and deglaze your pan so pleasantly that there will be almost no tidy up toward the finish of dinner as well.

Ingredients:

- 4 breast (daintily cut)
- Uncooked boneless skinless chicken breast
- Rosemary
- Table salt
- 2 tsp(s) (cleaved)
- Black pepper
- ½ tsp(s)
- ¼ tsp(s)
- 2 tsp(s)
- Uncooked shallot(s)
- Olive oil
- 2 item(s) (meagerly cut)
- 2 clove(s), medium (minced)
- Garlic clove(s)
- 2 tbsp(s)
- Fresh cherry tomato (es)
- Balsamic vinegar
- ¼ cup(s)
- Capers
- 2 tsp(s) (drained)
- Lemon zing

- 1 tbsp(s) (grated)
- 2 cup(s), red or yellow (or a blend of both), divided
- Fat free reduced sodium chicken stock

Method:

✓ Sprinkle chicken with 1/4 tsp salt, 1/2 tsp rosemary, and pepper. Heat oil in an enormous pan over medium-high heat. Add chicken and cook just until seared and cooked through, 2-3 minutes for every side. Move chicken to a platter and keep warm.

✓ Add shallots and garlic to a similar pan; cook over medium heat, mixing, until mollified, around 2 minutes. Add vinegar; cook, blending with a wooden spoon and scraping up any brown colored pieces from the lower part of the dish until vinegar vanishes.

✓ Mix in stock, escapades, tomatoes, lemon zing, staying 1/2 teaspoons rosemary, and staying 1/4 teaspoons salt. Cook, blending as often as possible until tomatoes are mollified, around 3 minutes. Return chicken and any gathered juices to pan; heat through.

Outrageous Herbacious Mediterranean Chickpea Salad

This basic chickpea salad is elevating, filling, and one of my outright most loved dinners to need to sit tight in my fridge for solid snacks. Made with ringer peppers, on the whole, fresh spices, fresh cucumber, and rich feta, each chomp tastes of warm, radiant minutes. Eating it never neglects to light up my mind-set. Protein-and fiber-rich chickpeas make it a generous vegan principle, or you can serve it as a simple side with chicken, fish, or shrimp.

Ingredients:

- Chickpeas
- Fresh parsley
- Red chime pepper
- Red onion
- Extra virgin olive oil
- Celery
- Lemon juice
- Genuine salt and pepper
- Garlic

Method:

- ✓ The main part of the recipe comes from canned chickpeas otherwise known as garbanzo beans, a staple I generally suggest having in the pantry. Essentially channel and wash and you're on your way.
- ✓ Add the chickpeas to a huge bowl close by the slashed ringer pepper, onion, parsley, and celery.

✓ Beat together the straightforward lemon dressing and pour over the chickpea combination. Throw to cover, then serve right away.

Mediterranean Stuffed Chicken Breasts

This Mediterranean Stuffed Chicken Breasts Recipe is simple, solid, and can be for the most part set up ahead of time. It freezes and warms well, as well, making it ideal for large clump cooking. Furthermore, it suits a variety of dietary recipes: low-carb, keto, gluten-free, and low-calorie. No big surprise it is likewise one of my #1 primary courses to serve when we have organization. The mix of nutty Parmesan and flavorful Mediterranean vegetables in a completely cooked chicken breast is stunning.

Ingredients:

- 1/4 cup disintegrated reduced-fat feta cheddar or 1 ounce disintegrated decreased fat feta cheddar
- 4 boneless skinless chicken breast parts or 1 - 1/2 lb boneless skinless chicken breast half
- 2 tablespoons finely slashed drained packaged roasted sweet red peppers
- 1/4 cup finely hacked drained packaged marinated artichoke hearts
- 2 tablespoons daintily cut green onions
- Nonstick cooking shower
- 1/8 teaspoon grated black pepper
- 2 teaspoons clipped fresh oregano or 1/2 teaspoon dried oregano, squashed

Method:

- ✓ Utilizing a sharp blade, cut a pocket in every chicken breast by slicing on a level recipe through the thickest bit too, however not through, the contrary side. Put in a safe spot.
- ✓ In a little bowl, join feta, artichoke hearts, cooked peppers, green onion, and oregano. Spoon uniformly into pockets in chicken breasts. If essential, secure openings with wooden toothpicks. Sprinkle chicken with black pepper.
- ✓ Coat an unheated huge nonstick pan with a cooking shower. Preheat pan over medium heat. Add chicken. Cook for 12 to 14 minutes or until not, at this point pink (170 degrees F), turning once.

Recipe: 15

Avocado Caprese Salad

Avocados are brimming with magnesium and potassium, they're the supplements that help diminish pulse. Tomatoes are loaded up with lycopene and help defeat colon disease. Arugula and basil are cell reinforcements and helps with maturing and convey hostile to cancer properties. Also, mozzarella... calcium, protein, and downright great.

Ingredients:

- 1 ea. Avocado from Mexico hollowed, stripped, and cut
- 2 ea. medium tomatoes, cut into 8 cuts
- 8 oz. fresh mozzarella, cut into 8 cuts
- 2 T. extra virgin olive oil
- 1 ea. pack of basil leaves isolated
- 1/8 t. pepper
- 1/8 t. salt

Method:

- ✓ On a huge serving platter, layer the cuts of tomato, avocado, mozzarella, and basil leaves, fanning them out marginally.
- ✓ Sprinkle with olive oil.
- ✓ Serve with salt and pepper.

Recipe: 16

Charred Shrimp & Pesto Buddha Bowls

These shrimp and pesto Buddha bowls are tasty, sound, and pretty and take under 30 minutes to prepare. At the end of the day, they're fundamentally a definitive simple weeknight dinner. Don't hesitate to add extra vegetables and trade the shrimp for chicken, steak, tofu, or edamame.

Ingredients:

- 2 tablespoons balsamic vinegar
- ⅓ cup arranged pesto
- 1 tablespoon extra-virgin olive oil
- ¼ teaspoon grated pepper
- ½ teaspoon salt
- 1 pound stripped and deveined huge shrimp (16-20 tally), wiped off
- 4 cups arugula
- 1 cup split cherry tomatoes
- 2 cups cooked quinoa
- 1 avocado, cubed

Method:

- ✓ Beat pesto, vinegar, oil, salt, and pepper in a huge bowl. Eliminate 4 tablespoons of the combination to a little bowl; put the two dishes in a safe spot.

- ✓ Heat an enormous cast-iron pan over medium-high heat. Add shrimp and cook, mixing, until just cooked through with a slight burn, 4 to 5 minutes. Eliminate to a plate.
- ✓ Add arugula and quinoa to the huge bowl with the vinaigrette and throw to cover. Split the arugula combination between 4 dishes. Top with tomatoes, avocado, and shrimp. Sprinkle each bowl with 1 tablespoon of the saved pesto combination.

Recipe: 17

Citrus Shrimp and Avocado Salad

This Citrus Shrimp and Avocado Salad is a light, reviving dish for summer and makes the ideal canapé, lunch, or dinner. You can even feast prep the shrimp for the in a hurry. To take your Citrus Shrimp and Avocado Salad with you, prep the shrimp in advance, store in an enormous holder, and essentially prepare it on top of blended greens toward the morning—lunch is served!

Ingredients:

- 1 c. Lemon juice
- 1 c. Shurfine Orange Juice
- ¼ c. Shurfine Olive Oil
- ¾ c. Shurfine Ketchup
- 1 t. Horseradish (or to taste)
- 1 c. Cleaved fresh cilantro
- 1 c. Meagerly cut red onion
- 2 huge avocados, stripped, pitted, and cut ¼"thick
- 1 lb. Shurfine Chef™s Net Cooked Shrimp, defrosted

Method:

- ✓ In a huge bowl consolidate orange and lemon juice, ketchup, olive oil, and horseradish.
- ✓ Add shrimp, onions, and cilantro and blend to join.

- ✓ Cover and refrigerate for a few hours. Channel shrimp combination.
- ✓ Mastermind avocado cuts on the lower part of the shallow serving bowl and orchestrate the combination on top. Serve right away.

Spanakorizo

Spanakopita is an exemplary Greek vegan dish made with spinach and rice. It is most likely one of the best customary Greek recipes since it's loaded with bunches of spinach, fresh spices, onions, and lemon.

Ingredients:

- ¼ cup extra-virgin olive oil
- 2.2 lb spinach, cleaned
- Salt, freshly grated pepper
- 1 onion, slashed
- 1 leek, slashed
- 1 ball green onions with leaves
- 1 tomato, cubed
- 1 ball fresh dill
- ¾ teacup Carolina rice
- Juice of 1 lemon

Method:

- ✓ Clean, flush, and channel the spinach completely. Generally, cleave.
- ✓ Heat the olive oil in a wide, shallow pot with a thick base (Rondeau) and sauté the onions, leek, and green onions for 3-4 minutes, until straightforward.
- ✓ Add the spinach, cubed tomatoes, and rice.
- ✓ Mix until gently shriveled and afterward add 1 ½ cups of water.

- ✓ Serve to taste and stew for 20 minutes.
- ✓ Sprinkle the cleaved dill towards the end, and pour in the lemon juice.
- ✓ Blend well and serve right away

Tsigareli

Tsigareli is elaborated with a sprinkle of olive oil. t is a well-known recipe. It can be delighted in as a side dish as well.

Ingredients:

- 2/3 cup olive oil
- 2 leeks, managed, daintily cut, washed well, and drained
- 10 to 12 green garlic stalks (white in addition to the vast majority of the green parts), daintily cut, or 4 enormous garlic cloves, coarsely cleaved
- 2 pounds' greens with stems (spinach and severe greens like dandelion and mustard greens; tawny and the external green leaves of any sort of lettuce like romaine, butterhead or green leaf; amaranth shoots and turnip greens; or broccoli rabe, Swiss chard, and frisée), leaves coarsely hacked, stems finely slashed
- 1 to 3 teaspoons Aleppo pepper or 1/2 - 1 teaspoon squashed red pepper drops
- 2 enormous ready tomatoes, cored and cubed, or 1 cup canned cubed tomatoes with their juice, or 1 cup water
- 1 teaspoon salt
- 1 1/2 cups bubbling water or chicken stock
- 1 cup coarsely hacked fresh level leaf parsley
- 1 cup coarsely slashed arugula
- Freshly grated black pepper
- Extra virgin olive oil to sprinkle (discretionary)
- 2 lemons, quartered (discretionary)
- For serving: cooked polenta, rice pilaf, or fresh dry bread

Method:

- ✓ In a big, profound pan, heat the oil and sauté the leeks and green garlic, if utilizing, for five to eight minutes, or until the leeks are delicate. If you are utilizing garlic cloves, add them now and cook briefly more.
- ✓ Add the stems of the greens and the Aleppo pepper or pepper chips. Sauté briefly, blending, then add the tomatoes or water and salt.
- ✓ Decrease the heat to low and stew for 10 minutes.
- ✓ Add the cook for 10 minutes.
- ✓ Add a large portion of a cup every one of the parsley and arugula and stews for eight minutes or more, until the greater part of the juices have vanished and the greens are delicate. If the sauce is as yet watery, cook for a couple of more minutes over high heat to lessen it.
- ✓ Mix in the leftover half cup every parsley and arugula, taste and change the flavors, adding a couple of toils of black pepper, and sprinkling with extra virgin olive oil if you like.
- ✓ Serve warm with the lemon wedges.

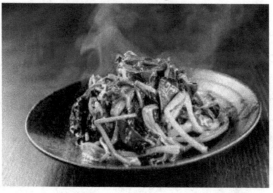

Falafel

Falafel is a tasty ball of chickpea and spice goodness that you find in Middle Eastern cooking. Normally veggie lover and vegan, falafel are incredible in wraps, pitas, sandwiches, and salads. Today, I'll share how to make both seared falafel and heated falafel. You pick your top choice!

Ingredients:

- 1 cup dried chickpeas
- 2 tablespoons finely hacked fresh parsley
- 1/2 huge onion, generally slashed (around 1 cup)
- 2 tablespoons finely hacked fresh cilantro
- 1/2-1 teaspoon dried hot red pepper
- 1 teaspoon salt
- 4 cloves of garlic
- 1 teaspoon heating powder
- 1 teaspoon cumin
- Soybean or vegetable oil for browning
- Pita bread
- 4-6 tablespoons flour
- Cleaved tomato for decorate
- Cubed green ringer pepper to decorate
- Cubed onion to decorate
- Tahina sauce

Method:

- ✓ Drench dried chickpeas short-term (truly, making sure to do this is the hardest part!)
- ✓ Barrage with spices, flavors, garlic, flour, and a hint of water
- ✓ Structure balls, refrigerate to solidify
- ✓ Fry until profound brilliant brown colored and very fresh

✓ Eat up as quick as humanly conceivable. Falafels are at their supreme pinnacle straight out of the fryer.

Lentil Soup with Kale

This lentil and kale soup is the ideal recipe. It's a veggie-lover, overflowing with fiber and protein and simple to make. It's a filling, fulfilling soup that doesn't leave you hungry later in the day. Lentil soup is made with generally storeroom ingredients however includes generous greens and a crush of lemon for splendid, fresh flavor. It's prepared with a couple of my number one flavors and a lot of freshly ground black pepper. Truly, it's the best lentil soup I've ever had.

Ingredients:

- 1 tablespoon olive oil
- 1 cup water
- 1 huge sweet onion, sliced
- 4 medium carrots, stripped and hacked (around 1 ½ cups)
- 2 cloves garlic, minced
- 2 teaspoons fresh thyme leaves
- ¼ teaspoon squashed red pepper chips (pretty much to taste)
- 4 cups vegetable stock
- ⅓ Cup dry red lentils washed
- 1 (6-ounce) would tomato be able to glue
- ⅓ Cup dry green or Puy lentils, flushed
- 1 tablespoon brown colored sugar
- ½ teaspoon garam masala
- 1 tablespoon white vinegar
- 1 teaspoon fresh ground black pepper
- 2 tablespoons minced fresh parsley
- 3 cups kale leaves, stems eliminated, cut into reduced down pieces

Method:

- ✓ Pour the olive oil into an enormous Dutch stove or soup pot. Heat on medium-high until the oil is gleaming. Add the carrots and onion.
- ✓ Sauté for 5 minutes, or until the vegetables are fresh delicate.
- ✓ Add the garlic, squashed red pepper, and thyme leaves. Sauté until the garlic is fragrant, around 1 moment.
- ✓ Add the vegetable stock, water, and lentils to the pot. Heat to the point of boiling. Diminish the heat, cover, and stew for 25 to 30 minutes.
- ✓ Add every excess ingredient: tomato glue, vinegar, brown colored sugar, garam masala, pepper, kale, and parsley. Return the soup to a bubble, then decrease the heat and cook, revealed, for 10 minutes or until the kale is shriveled.
- ✓ Present with a scramble of hot sauce, whenever wanted. Enhancement with parsley.

Recipe: 22

Mediterranean Ravioli with Artichokes & Olives

The center of a Mediterranean diet dinner plan is comprised of food sources from plant sources structure, while food sources from creature sources structure the periphery. Exploration recommends that the Mediterranean Ravioli with Artichokes and Olives would be defensive against persistent sickness. Mediterranean Ravioli with Artichokes and Olives is an advantageous and fundamental piece of the Mediterranean eating routine and ought to be viewed as except if it would put a person in danger.

Ingredients:

- ½ cup oil-stuffed sun-dried tomatoes, depleted (2 tablespoons oil saved)
- 2 (8 ounces) bundles of frozen or refrigerated spinach-and-ricotta ravioli
- 1 (10 ounces) bundle frozen quartered artichoke hearts, defrosted
- ¼ cup Kalamata olives, cut
- 1 (15 ounces) can no-salt-added cannellini beans, washed
- ¼ cup fresh basil
- 3 tablespoons toasted pine nuts

Method:

- ✓ Boil a big pot of water. Cook ravioli as indicated by bundle bearings. Channel and throw with 1 tablespoon held oil; put in a safe spot.
- ✓ Heat the excess 1 tablespoon oil in an enormous nonstick skillet over medium heat. Add artichokes and beans; sauté until warmed through, 2 to 3 minutes.
- ✓ Crease in the cooked ravioli, pine nuts, olives, sun-dried tomatoes, and basil.

Recipe: 23

Easy Couscous with Sun-Dried Tomato and Feta

Couscous Salad with sun-dried tomato, feta, rocket (arugula), spices, and the nutty wonderfulness of chickpeas. My easy route flavor tip is to utilize the oil from the sun-dried tomato container as the dressing–free flavor. For a fast scrumptious salad recipe, you can't go past this one. It's fresh, delicious, and will dazzle your loved ones. You can make it early and it endures truly well in the refrigerator, without the feta and rocket, which can be added at the hour of serving.

Ingredients:

- 1 red pepper, cultivated and cubed
- 175g couscous
- 1 teaspoon ground cumin
- 1/3 cucumber, cultivated and cubed
- 3 tablespoons olive oil
- 3 tablespoons lemon juice
- 10 sun-dried tomatoes, hacked
- 2 tablespoons freshly hacked mint

Method:

- ✓ Cook the couscous as per the directions on the parcel; move into an enormous salad bowl.
- ✓ Add cubed red pepper, cucumber, and sun-dried tomatoes to couscous; blend well.
- ✓ Beat olive oil, lemon juice, sliced mint, and ground cumin together in a little bowl.
- ✓ Pour dressing over couscous; throw well and sprinkle disintegrated feta cheddar on top.
- ✓ Serve to taste with salt and freshly ground black pepper.

Recipe: 24

Vegan Mediterranean Lentil Soup

There are countless plans in the Mediterranean locale on the best way to cook Lentil Soup. This particular recipe is common on Fresh Year's Eve since it represents wealth from the lentils. However, I will cook it for my family any possibility I get. Mediterranean Lentil Soup is fit as a fiddle comfort food, particularly on a cool day.

Ingredients:

- 2 cups hacked onion
- 1 tablespoon olive oil
- 1 teaspoon ground turmeric

- 1 teaspoon stew powder
- 1 teaspoon ground cumin
- 1/4 teaspoon salt
- 1/4 teaspoon black pepper
- 1 teaspoon ground red pepper
- 2 garlic cloves, minced
- 2 1/3 cups dried lentils
- 3 1/3 cups water
- 1/3 cup fresh cilantro
- 1 (28-ounce) can cubed tomatoes, undrained
- 3 (14 1/2-ounce) jars without fat, less-sodium chicken stock, or meat stock (I incline toward hamburger some favor chicken)
- 2 tablespoons red wine vinegar
- 1 or 2 Bay leaves

Optional:

- Sliced fresh tomatoes (optional)
- For embellish (top each bowl with)
- Cilantro branch (optional)

Method:

- ✓ Heat olive oil in an enormous Dutch broiler over medium-high heat.
- ✓ Add the onion; sauté for 3 minutes or until delicate.
- ✓ Add the turmeric and the following 6 ingredients (turmeric through garlic); sauté for 1 moment.
- ✓ Add water and next 4 ingredients (water through cubed tomatoes); add cove leaf and heat to the point of boiling. Diminish heat; stew for 60 minutes. sprinkle with red wine vinegar optional:
- ✓ Hold 2 cups of lentil combination.

- ✓ Spot half of the excess combination in a blender; measure until smooth.
- ✓ Pour pureed soup into a huge bowl.
- ✓ Rehash the system with another portion of the excess combination.
- ✓ Mix in held 2 cups lentil combination.
- ✓ Topping with sliced tomatoes and a cilantro ranch, whenever wanted.

Recipe: 25

Greek Salad with Avocado

Avocado Greek salad with a Greek salad dressing is a family most loved side salad presented with anything. A contort on the customary Greek Salad! Stacked up with rich avocado and a hint of lettuce alongside green peppers (or capsicum), tomatoes, cucumbers, feta, olives, and onion. The best side salad for any supper!

Ingredients:

- 4 enormous tomatoes cut into more modest pieces
- 1/4 medium red onion cut or slashed
- 4 Persian (scaled down) cucumbers (or one entire English cucumber) cut
- 2 avocados slashed
- 1 green pepper slashed
- Kalamata olives to taste
- 7-ounce feta cubed
- Salt and pepper to taste

Dressing:

- 1 teaspoon dried oregano
- 2 teaspoons red wine vinegar
- 3 tablespoons olive oil

- 1 teaspoon lemon juice

Method:

- ✓ Prep the tomatoes, cucumbers, red onion, avocados, green pepper, feta, and olives and add them to an enormous salad bowl.
- ✓ Beat together the dressing ingredients in a little bowl
- ✓ Prepare the salad. You may have to change the oil/vinegar amounts to suit your taste. I like to add some salt and pepper even though the feta and olives are genuinely pungent.
- ✓ Sprinkle some extra dried oregano over the top preceding serving whenever wanted.

Recipe: 26

EatingWell's Eggplant Parmesan

Eggplant Parmesan doesn't need to incorporate layers of roasted eggplant and piles of cheddar. This solid eggplant Parmesan recipe has is fulfilling without heaping on the calories and fat. Try not to avoid the progression of salting the eggplant, particularly if you need to freeze one of the goulashes. Salting assists with drawing out the additional dampness so the eggplant holds up better in the cooler. Present with a salad of unpleasant greens threw with a red-wine vinaigrette.

Ingredients:

- 3 egg whites
- 2 eggplants, (around 2 pounds all-out)
- 3 tablespoons water
- 1 cup fine dry breadcrumbs
- ½ teaspoon salt
- 1/2 cup freshly ground Parmesan cheddar, (1 ounce), isolated
- ½ teaspoon freshly ground pepper
- 2 ½ cups pureed tomatoes
- ¼ cup fragmented fresh basil leaves

- 3/4 cup ground part-skim mozzarella cheddar, (3 ounces)

Method:

- ✓ Position racks in the center and lower thirds of the stove; preheat to 400°F. Coat 2 heating sheets and a 9-by-13-inch preparing dish with a cooking shower.
- ✓ Beat eggs and water in a shallow bowl. Blend breadcrumbs, 1/4 cup Parmesan and Italian flavoring in another shallow dish. Plunge eggplant in the egg combination, then covers with the breadcrumb blend, tenderly squeezing to follow.
- ✓ Mastermind the eggplant in a solitary layer on the readied heating sheets. Liberally splash the two sides of the eggplant with a cooking shower. Heat, flipping the eggplant and exchanging the container between racks most of the way until the eggplant is delicate and softly caramelized around 30 minutes. Serve with salt and pepper.
- ✓ Then, blend pureed tomatoes, basil, garlic, and squashed red pepper in a medium bowl.
- ✓ Spread around 1/2 cup of the sauce in the readied heating dish. Orchestrate a large portion of the eggplant cuts over the sauce.
- ✓ Spoon over 1 cup sauce on the eggplant.
- ✓ Sprinkle with 1/2 cup mozzarella and 1/4 cup Parmesan.
- ✓ Top with the sauce, eggplant, and cheddar.
- ✓ Prepare until the sauce is percolating and the top is brilliant for 20 to 30 minutes. Let cool for 5 minutes. Sprinkle with more basil before serving, whenever wanted.

Autumn Cous Salad

Make proper acquaintance with butternut squash and fall flavors contacted by a tart pucker in my tribute to Whole Foods Market's Autumn Couscous Salad. This pre-winter couscous salad is a bright festival of the period, studded with the very most awesome aspect of fall's abundance. This salad could be served warm, yet I lean toward it actually like on the salad bar, or at room temperature, and it just improves the more extended the flavors have the opportunity to merge.

Ingredients:

- 591 ml butternut squash
- 355 ml squeezed apple
- 1 shallot
- 59.1 ml oil
- 118 ml dried currants
- 177 ml improved dried cranberries
- 1 fennel bulbs
- 6 servings coarse genuine salt
- 3 tbsp sage leaves
- 1 tbsp unadulterated olive oil
- 227 g dry pearl couscous
- 1 tbsp parsley leaves
- 3 tbsps. red wine vinegar

Method:

✓ Get water to heat a medium-size pot, add couscous, and heat back to the point of boiling then lower to medium, and cook until still somewhat firm, around 8 minutes.

- ✓ Channel in a colander, yet don't wash. Put to the side in a blending bowl to cool.
- ✓ Heat olive oil in an enormous sauté dish over medium-high heat.
- ✓ Add the shallot and cook for 1 moment, blending frequently.
- ✓ Add cubed fennel and cook for an additional 5 minutes or until fennel relaxes.
- ✓ Add butternut squash, sage, cranberries, currants, and squeezed apple and cook for 15 minutes or until butternut squash has relaxed and practically the entirety of the squeezed apple has cooked down. Serve with legitimate salt and pepper.
- ✓ Move the combination to the bowl with the couscous, saving about ¼ cup of the squeezed apple for the vinaigrette. In a little bowl, blend the held squeezed apple, canola oil, red wine vinegar, and more salt and pepper to taste.
- ✓ Add to the couscous with the parsley and mix.
- ✓ Allow couscous to sit at room temperature for around 30 minutes for flavors to merge before serving.

Recipe: 28

Tuscan Tuna and White Bean Salad

The Tuscan Tuna and White Bean Salad are too sound and stacked with Mediterranean flavors. If you battle with getting sufficient protein in your diet check this simple-to-make salad out. It utilizes straightforward ingredients to make a stunning dinner. I suggest utilizing quality fish since it is the genuine star of the dish.

Ingredients:

- 1/2 c. daintily cut red onion divided
- 1 can white cannellini beans
- 1 can fish (6 oz) in olive oil, channel, and save oil
- 1/2 c. pitted kalamata olives
- 1 cup cubed plum tomatoes

- 2 tbsp. hacked Italian parsley
- 1/2 tsp. ground lemon zing
- 1/4 tsp salt
- 1/4 tsp black pepper
- 1 tbsp. lemon juice
- 4 thick flatbreads
- 2 cups torn arugula leaves

Method:

- ✓ In a bowl, fish, consolidate beans, lemon zing, tomatoes, red onion, olives, olive oil, parsley, lemon squeeze, salt, and pepper.
- ✓ Throw tenderly to consolidate and add arugula
- ✓ Preheat flame broil or barbecue dish.
- ✓ Brush flatbreads daintily with the leftover-held olive oil.
- ✓ Barbecue until softly caramelized around 2 mins for every side.
- ✓ Cut flatbreads in equal parts or quarters. Present with a salad.

Recipe: 29

Prosciutto Pizza with Corn & Arugula

Prosciutto and arugula lift this basic barbecued pizza. If you have time, let the batter remain at room temperature for 10 to 15 minutes to make carrying it out simpler in this 20-minute sound pizza recipe.

Ingredients:

- 2 tablespoons extra-virgin olive oil, partitioned
- 1-pound pizza batter, ideally entire wheat
- 1 clove garlic, minced
- 1 cup fresh corn pieces
- 1 cup part-skim destroyed mozzarella cheddar
- 1 ounce meagerly cut prosciutto, attacked 1-inch pieces
- 1/2 cup torn fresh basil
- 1/2 cups arugula
- 1/4 teaspoon ground pepper

Method:

- ✓ Preheat flame broil to medium-high.
- ✓ Carry mixture out on a softly floured surface into a 12-inch oval.
- ✓ Move to a daintily floured enormous preparing sheet.
- ✓ Consolidate 1 tablespoon oil and garlic in a little bowl. Bring the butter, garlic oil, cheddar, corn, and prosciutto to the flame broil.
- ✓ Oil the barbecue rack.
- ✓ Move the outside layer to the barbecue.
- ✓ Barbecue the batter until puffed and gently cooked for 1 to 2 minutes.
- ✓ Flip the outside layer over and spread the garlic oil on it.
- ✓ Top with cheddar, corn, and prosciutto.
- ✓ Flame broil, covered until the cheddar is liquefied and the outside layer is gently caramelized on the last, 2 to 3 minutes more. Return the pizza to the heating sheet.
- ✓ Top the pizza with arugula, basil, and pepper. Sprinkle with the excess 1 tablespoon oil.

Recipe: 30

Garlicky Swiss Chard and Chickpeas

This is one of those go-to dishes for occupied weeknights—it's quick, simple, and filling. It additionally turns out to be a veggie lover recipe where vegetables and entire grains become the dominant focal point. Heaps of garlic assemble an appetizing flavor base, while Swiss chard contributes a strongly hearty flavor.

In case you're not a major devotee of chard, you can likewise substitute a milder green, for example, spinach or infant kale. For heartier cravings, have a go at garnish each presenting with a singed or poached egg. What's more, that reminds us—however, we're calling this supper, it would likewise be unbelievable for breakfast.

Ingredients:

- 2 packs Swiss chard, focus stems cut out and disposed of and leaves coarsely sliced
- 1 tablespoon olive oil, partitioned
- 2 medium shallots, finely sliced (about ½ cup)6 medium garlic cloves, minced
- 2 cups low-sodium chicken stock (or vegetable stock)
- 15.5 ounce can garbanzo beans (chickpeas), flushed and depleted
- Salt and freshly ground black pepper, to taste
- 2 tablespoons freshly crushed lemon juice
- ½ cup disintegrated feta cheddar, optional

Method:

- ✓ In a huge skillet, heat 1 tablespoon of olive oil over medium-high heat.
- ✓ Add half chard and cook it for 1 - 2 minutes.
- ✓ When the principal half has withered, add the leftover chard.
- ✓ When the entirety of the chard is withered, add the chicken stock.
- ✓ Cover the skillet and cook the chard until delicate, around 10 minutes. Channel the chard through a fine (sifter) and put it in a safe spot.
- ✓ Crash the skillet and heat the leftover 1 tablespoon olive oil over medium-high heat.
- ✓ Add the shallots and garlic and cook, mixing, until they are relaxed, around 2 minutes.
- ✓ Add the chard and chickpeas and cook until warmed through 3 to 4 minutes.
- ✓ Sprinkle the lemon juice over the blend and serve with salt and pepper, to taste.
- ✓ Sprinkle cheddar on top not long before serving, whenever wanted.

Chicken Parmesan-Stuffed Spaghetti Squash

This filling, good stuffed spaghetti squash is a lower-carb variant of your conventional chicken Parmesan with pasta. This chicken Parmesan recipe is still loaded with messy goodness, however, has the additional advantage of sweet winter squash. If you can't discover two little squashes, use one (3-pound) squash and cut every half into two bits when prepared to serve.

Ingredients:

- Huge Spaghetti Squash
- 2 Eggs/beaten
- 2 Boneless Skinless Chicken Breasts/cut into strips
- Flour
- Marinara Sauce
- Italian Style Breadcrumbs
- Oil for broiling
- Destroyed Mozzarella Cheese
- Italian Serving
- Salt
- Ground Parmesan Cheese
- Pepper

Method:

✓ With a sharp blade, cut the squash into equal parts. (If the squash is excessively intense - cut in a few spots shaping a specked line around the squash. Microwave for 3-5 minutes to relax. Permit to cool before slicing down the middle - following the spotted line).

✓ Scoop out the seeds - brush with oil, salt, and pepper, - and cook face down in a preheated broiler at 375°F (190°C) for 35-40 minutes (until a fork can undoubtedly penetrate the skin).

✓ In the interim, cut the chicken bosoms into strips. Spot flour, beaten egg, and breadcrumbs into three separate dishes. Coat each strip with flour, then egg, and afterward move in bread morsels.

✓ Heat a very much oiled skillet over medium/high heat. Fry the chicken fingers (in clumps if important) until brilliant brown colored on all sides and cooked through. Put to the side on paper towels.

✓ When the squash has completed the process of broiling - eliminate it from the stove and let it set for a couple of moments before turning over and pulling at it with a fork. Shred within each squash, being mindful so as not to jab through the skin.

✓ Pour marinara sauce over destroyed squash. Top with chicken tenders, then more marinara, and get done with mozzarella and Parmesan cheddar, and a touch of Italian flavoring. Get back to the stove to heat for 10-15 minutes until the cheddar has dissolved. Appreciate!

Recipe: 32

Green Shakshuka with Spinach, Chard & Feta

In Israel, the best and ideal opportunity to make this shakshuka is in the colder time of year when spinach, chard, and other verdant greens are at their best. Thick, marginally tart stews produced using moderately cooked greens are one of the signs of both Tunisian and Libyan food. So if red shakshuka were made with extra tomato stews, it's altogether conceivable that extra stews of stewed greens were repurposed as green shakshuka.

Ingredients:

- 1/4 cup (60 mL) extra-virgin olive oil
- 2 leeks, white parts hacked and green tops daintily cut
- 3 medium garlic cloves, meagerly cut
- 1 little jalapeño stew, cored, cultivated, and meagerly cut
- 5 or 6 Swiss chard leaves, leaves coarsely hacked, stems meagerly cut
- 1 little pack Tuscan kale (additionally called lacinato or dinosaur), stemmed, leaves coarsely cleaved
- 3 cups infant spinach or managed and coarsely slashed standard spinach
- 1 tsp (5 mL) ground caraway
- 1 tsp (5 mL) ground cumin
- Fit salt and freshly ground black pepper
- 1/2 cup (120 mL) natively constructed or low-sodium locally acquired chicken stock or vegetable stock or water
- 1 tbsp (15 mL) fresh lemon juice
- 6 to 8 huge eggs

Method:

- ✓ Heat the oil in a big skillet (over medium heat). Add the leeks, garlic, jalapeño, and chard stems and sauté until mollified and daintily caramelized, 10 to 12 minutes (take care not to brown the garlic).
- ✓ Add the kale, spinach, and chard leaves and cook, mixing regularly, until withered and delicate, 3 to 4 minutes. Add the caraway and cumin, and serve softly with salt (the feta is very pungent) and a few spots of pepper.
- ✓ Add the stock and the lemon squeeze and cook for 5 to 7 minutes, then decrease the heat to low and cook for an additional couple of moments, until the greens merge into a thick, dim green, stewy sauce. Taste and change the flavoring.
- ✓ Use a huge spoon to make little wells in the greens blend. Cautiously break 1 egg into a cup or ramekin, then slip it into one of the wells; rehash with the leftover eggs.
- ✓ Cover and stew until the egg whites are set however the yolks are still a little runny, around 7 minutes. Eliminate the skillet from the heat.
- ✓ Sprinkle the shakshuka with the feta, shower with oil, and sprinkle liberally with za'atar. Serve the shakshuka straightforwardly from the skillet, with a lot of hard bread or challah.

Recipe: 33

Chicken Caprese Sandwich

For those of you in a comparable circumstance, take a stab at preparing Open Face Chicken Caprese Sandwiches for a fast and simple supper on a feverish Wednesday (or any working day) night. They're inconceivably delectable, filling, and, most amazing aspect all, prepared in only 15 minutes.

This Stuffed Chicken Caprese Sandwich is our number one summer barbecue recipe! Chicken bosoms loaded down with fresh mozzarella, basil, and tomato, marinated in balsamic decrease, barbecued, and made into a scrumptious chicken sandwich.

Ingredients:

- 3 tbsp olive oil
- 4 boneless skinless chicken bosom parts
- 3 tbsp balsamic vinegar
- 1/2 tsp salt
- 2 cloves garlic, minced
- 1/4 tsp pepper
- 2 tbsp olive oil
- 8 cuts bread
- 8-ounce fresh mozzarella, cut
- 1/2 cup fresh basil leaves
- 8 tomato cuts
- balsamic decrease, natively constructed or locally acquired

Method:

- ✓ In a little bowl, beat together olive oil, balsamic vinegar, minced garlic, salt, and pepper.
- ✓ Spot chicken bosoms in a preparing dish and cover them with marinade. Refrigerate in any event 30 minutes, up to expedite.
- ✓ Preheat flame broil to medium-high heat.
- ✓ Flame broil the chicken bosoms for 5-7 minutes on each side, contingent upon the thickness until interior temperature peruses 165 degrees F.
- ✓ Brush cuts of bread with olive oil.
- ✓ Barbecue each piece 1-2 minutes on each side.
- ✓ To collect sandwiches, place one chicken bosom half on a cut of bread.
- ✓ Top with mozzarella cheddar, tomato cuts, and basil leaves.
- ✓ Sprinkle with balsamic decrease and afterward top with a cut of bread.
- ✓ Serve and appreciate!

Shakshuka

Shakshuka might be at the summit of eggs-for-supper plans, however in Israel, it is a breakfast food, a splendid, fiery beginning to the day with a heap of pita or challah served as an afterthought. (It likewise makes superb informal breakfast or lunch food.) It's a one-skillet recipe of eggs prepared in a tomato-red pepper sauce spiced with cumin, paprika, and cayenne.

Shakshuka started in North Africa, and like numerous extraordinary dishes, there are however many forms as there are cooks who have accepted it. This one wanderer from more customary versions by adding disintegrated feta cheddar, which mollifies into smooth pieces in the broiler's heat.

Ingredients:

- 1/2 onion, cleaved
- 1/2 tablespoons extra-virgin olive oil
- 1/2 red ringer pepper, meagerly cut
- 2 little cloves garlic, daintily cut
- 1/2 teaspoon paprika
- 3/4 teaspoon ground cumin
- Squeeze red pepper pieces
- 4 huge eggs
- Genuine salt and freshly ground pepper
- Warm pita bread, for serving
- 1 15-ounce can entire stripped tomatoes, squashed by hand
- 1/4 little bundle cilantro, leaves, and delicate stems isolated slashed

Method:

- ✓ Heat the olive oil in a skillet.
- ✓ Add the onion and chime pepper and cook, blending at times, until delicate, around 10 minutes.
- ✓ Add the cilantro stems, garlic, cumin, paprika, and red pepper pieces; serve with 1/4 teaspoon salt and a couple of toils of pepper.
- ✓ Cook, blending until the garlic is relaxed and the vegetables are covered with the flavors, around 1 moment.
- ✓ Preheat the broiler to 375 degrees F. Mix the tomatoes with their juices into the skillet.
- ✓ Lessen the heat to keep a low stew and cook, blending incidentally, until the tomatoes separate and the sauce thickens somewhat, around 20 minutes; serve with salt and pepper.
- ✓ Use the rear of a spoon to make 4 wells in the sauce, 1 to 2 inches separated. Break an egg into each well.
- ✓ Run the edge of an elastic spatula through the egg whites to break them somewhat, being mindful so as not to break the yolks (this permits the egg whites to cook quicker).
- ✓ Move the skillet to the broiler and heat until the egg whites are simply set, 15 to 18 minutes. Serve with salt and pepper and top with cilantro leaves. Present with pita bread.

Recipe: 35

Eggplant Frittata

This frankfurter and eggplant frittata is intended for summer informal breakfasts or simple weeknight dinners, served warm or at room temperature. Meltingly delicate eggplant and a stack of basil make it taste like the serve, while zesty wiener and velvety goat cheddar beef it up.

Ingredients:

- 2 tablespoons coarsely slashed fresh dill
- Fit salt
- 2 little eggplants (around 7 ounces each), stripped and cut into 1/4-inch dice
- 1/4 cup olive oil
- 1 dozen enormous eggs
- 2 medium onions, daintily cut
- Freshly ground pepper

Method:

- ✓ Preheat the broiler to 350°. Put the eggplant in a colander and throw with 1 teaspoon of genuine salt.
- ✓ Spot a little plate on top of the eggplant and burden it with canned products.
- ✓ Set the colander in the sink until the eggplant delivers its fluid, around 30 minutes. Delicately crush the eggplant to eliminate extra dampness.
- ✓ In a huge ovenproof skillet, ideally nonstick, heat 2 tablespoons of olive oil. Add a large portion of the eggplant and cook over tolerably high heat, mixing sometimes, until caramelized, around 4 minutes.

- ✓ Move the eggplant to a huge plate and rehash it with the excess olive oil and eggplant.
- ✓ Decrease the heat to low, add the onion and cook until delicate, around 6 minutes. Return the eggplant to the skillet.
- ✓ In the interim, in a huge bowl, beat the eggs with a squeeze of every one of salt and pepper. Add the eggs to the eggplant and onion in the skillet and increment the heat to direct.
- ✓ When the frittata is generally set, tenderly mix in the dill. Put the skillet in the broiler and cook the frittata until it is simply set around 5 minutes.
- ✓ Shake the skillet to slacken the frittata and run a spatula around it if vital. Cautiously slide the frittata onto a platter, then let cool marginally.
- ✓ Cut into 12 wedges
- ✓ Serve hot.

Recipe: 36

Sweet Potato Toast

Allow me to acquaint you with my fresh most loved alternative Sweet Potato Toast! This healthy, gluten-free "toast", is absurdly simple to plan, and you can get truly inventive with the garnishes to keep every early daytime fascinating.

Sweet potato "toast" isn't crunchy like genuine toast and it won't trick anybody into believing that they're eating bread, yet it's thoroughly fulfilling in its specific manner. Truly, it's simply huge sweet potato cuts that are cooked until delicate, however not soft, so they are sufficiently healthy to hold your #1 toast garnishes.

Ingredients:

- 1 huge sweet potato

Method:

- ✓ Preheat the stove to 400ºF and fix a heating sheet with material paper to help forestall staying.
- ✓ Cut the finishes of the sweet potato off, then cut it the long way into 1/2-inch thick cuts. Organize the cuts in a solitary layer on the preparing sheet. (No oil required!)
- ✓ Heat until the cuts are delicate and effortlessly punctured with a fork, around 20 minutes. Serve warm with your #1 toast garnishes.
- ✓ Store any extra sweet potato cuts in an impenetrable compartment in the ice chest for as long as seven days. To warm for a simple breakfast pop, them in the toaster oven! (I use 3 out of 5 settings on my toaster oven.) Top and appreciate once more!

Recipe: 37

Arugula Salad with Pesto Shrimp, Parmesan and White Beans

This arugula plate of mixed greens is made with white beans, tomatoes, red onion, shaved parmesan cheddar, and pine nuts, all threw in a lemon dressing. A splendid and energetic salad that makes the ideal side dish or lighter primary course.

Ingredients:

- 4 tablespoons olive oil (separated)
- 2 cloves garlic (squeezed)
- 1/2-pound Simple Truth crude large shrimp
- 1/4 teaspoon freshly ground black pepper
- Touch of red pepper pieces

- 1/4 teaspoon legitimate salt
- 1/4 cup Hemisphares pesto
- 8 cups Simple Truth child arugula
- 2 cups Private Selection cherry tomatoes
- 1/2 lemon
- 1/2 cup canned Simple Truth cannellini or another white bean
- 1/8 cup freshly shaved Parmesan cheddar

Method:

- ✓ Whenever frozen, defrost the shrimp under cool water, filter, and wipe off with a paper towel, then place in a bowl.
- ✓ Shower with olive oil and throw with the garlic, fit salt, black pepper, and red pepper drops. Put in a safe spot for the flavors to merge for 20-30 minutes.
- ✓ Heat a non-stick skillet over medium-high heat. Shower the dish with 1 tablespoon of olive oil and add the shrimp each in turn, cautious not to stuff the skillet, cooking in two bunches.
- ✓ Cook for 2 minutes on one side, then flip the shrimp and cook just until murky, then move to a bowl.
- ✓ Diminish the heat marginally and add the remainder of the shrimp and the entirety of the oil and garlic from the bowl alongside the tomatoes to the skillet.
- ✓ Cook for 4-5 minutes, flipping the shrimp partially through and turning the tomatoes and garlic so the garlic doesn't consume and get severe.
- ✓ Take the skillet off the heat and move the shrimp to the bowl with the remainder of the cooked shrimp and throw with the pesto, and put in a safe spot.
- ✓ Add the arugula to a bowl, shower with the leftover olive oil, a liberal press of lemon squeeze, and throw with your fingers to cover.
- ✓ Cutthe Parmesan over the arugula

- ✓ Top with the beans, and the tomatoes.
- ✓ Serve with more genuine salt and freshly ground black pepper to taste and gobble it up.

Recipe: 38

Green Shakshuka

Green shakshuka puts a healthy green twist on the exemplary shakshuka recipe. It's a simple, one-container dish loaded up with shaved brussels sprouts, spinach, zucchini, and poached eggs. Regardless of whether you have it for breakfast or supper, it's a good, supplement-pressed dinner that will last you through any serve.

The incredible thing about a shakshuka is its flexibility. Like how you can throw most ingredients from your refrigerator into a smoothie, the equivalent can be said for a shakshuka.

Ingredients:

- 1 leek, pale area just, meagerly cut
- 1 tbs olive oil
- 1/2 tsp ground cumin
- 250g pkt frozen spinach, just defrosted, overabundance fluid eliminated
- 1/2 tsp smoked paprika
- 300ml light thickened cream
- 200g sugar snap peas, managed
- 1/2 cups (180g) frozen peas
- 100g depleted Persian fetta, disintegrated
- 4 Coles Australian Free Range Eggs
- Stew sauce, to serve

Method:

- ✓ Heat the oil in a skillet on average heat. Add the leek and cook, mixing, for 5 mins or until the leek relax.

- ✓ Add the cumin and paprika and cook for 1 min or until fragrant.
- ✓ Add spinach and cream to the dish. Cook, mixing, for 1-2 mins or until warmed through. Add the peas and sugar snap peas. Bring to a stew.
- ✓ Use the rear of an enormous metal spoon to make 4 huge indents in the pea blend. Cautiously break an egg into each indent.
- ✓ Cook, in part, covered, for 5 mins for delicate yolks or until the eggs are cooked as you would prefer. Eliminate from heat and sprinkle with the fetta. Shower with the bean stew sauce.

Caprese Stuffed Portobello Mushrooms

Caprese Stuffed Portobello Mushrooms topped with mozzarella, tomato, and fresh basil make for a delicious and nutritious tidbit or side dish! These exemplary flavors are ideal for serving a staggering however basic canapé for visitors or a treat for your family.

The kind of mushroom that we can discover here that is nearest to porcini is presumably the portobello assortment. These huge mushroom covers are substantial in flavor and are extraordinary stuffed. This is one more direct recipe that can be arranged in minutes yet is adequately rich to serve while engaging as a first course.

Ingredients:

- 1 cup fresh basil
- 12 ounces portobello mushrooms
- 1 tablespoon almonds
- 3 tablespoons margarine, dissolved
- 3 cloves garlic
- Cherry tomatoes cut down the middle and cultivated
- 3 tablespoons ground parmesan
- Fresh mozzarella gems

Method:

- ✓ Clean the mushrooms and eliminate the stems. Spot, cap side down into a heating dish.
- ✓ Preheat broiler to 400 degrees F.
- ✓ Spot the basil, almonds, and garlic into a scaled-down food processor and interact until little and uniform. Mix in the liquefied margarine and parmesan cheddar.

- ✓ Spread the basil combination into the cavities of the mushrooms. Top with a mozzarella pearl and a large portion of a cherry tomato.
- ✓ Heat in the preheated broiler for 15 minutes or until the mushrooms are starting to deliver their fluid and cheddar is softened. Whenever wanted, sear for 1 moment or brown colored the cheddar and tomatoes.
- ✓ Whenever wanted, embellish the fresh basil and serve

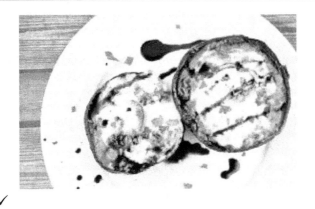

✓

Zucchini Lasagna Rolls with Smoked Mozzarella

Zucchini Rollatini is a tasty, messy, veggie-stacked dish! Made with pieces of barbecued zucchini loaded down with a basil-cheddar filling, then rolled and finished off with marinara, mozzarella, and prepared in the broiler until the cheddar is hot and softened.

Ingredients:

- 2 teaspoons extra-virgin olive oil
- 2 enormous zucchinis, managed
- ½ teaspoon ground pepper, isolated
- 8 tablespoons destroyed smoked mozzarella cheddar, isolated
- ¼ teaspoon salt, isolated
- 3 tablespoons ground Parmesan cheddar, isolated
- 1⅓ cups part-skim ricotta
- 1 enormous egg, delicately beaten
- 1 clove garlic, minced
- 1 (10 ounces) bundle frozen spinach, defrosted and pressed dry
- 2 tablespoons cleaved fresh basil
- ¾ cup low-sodium marinara sauce, partitioned

Method:

- ✓ Position racks in upper and lower thirds of broiler; preheat to 425 degrees F. Coat 2 rimmed preparing sheets with cooking shower.
- ✓ Cut zucchini longwise to get 24 all-out strips, around 1/8 inch thick each.
- ✓ Throw the zucchini, oil, 1/4 teaspoon pepper, and 1/8 teaspoon salt in a huge bowl. Mastermind the zucchini in single layers on the readied dish.
- ✓ Heat the zucchini, turning once, until delicate, around 10 minutes' aggregate.
- ✓ In the meantime, conhealthyate 2 tablespoons mozzarella and 1 tablespoon Parmesan in a little bowl.
- ✓ Blend egg, ricotta, spinach, garlic, and the excess 6 tablespoons mozzarella, 2 tablespoons Parmesan, 1/4 teaspoon pepper, and 1/8 teaspoon salt in a medium bowl.
- ✓ Spread 1/4 cup marinara in an 8-inch-square preparing dish. Spot 1 tablespoon of the ricotta combination close to the lower part of a segment of zucchini. Move it up and place, crease side down, in the preparing dish.
- ✓ Rehash with the excess zucchini and filling. Top the moves with the excess 1/2 cup marinara sauce and sprinkle with the saved cheddar blend.
- ✓ Prepare the zucchini moves until effervescent and gently cooked on top, around 20 minutes. Let represent 5 minutes. Sprinkle with basil before serving.

Kale and Butternut Squash Frittata

This kale butternut squash frittata is extraordinary for any dinner and can be eaten hot, cold, or in a hurry. This is an incredible method to get in verdant greens and a high protein feast that keeps well in the refrigerator.

Ingredients:

- 1 Tablespoon olive oil
- 4 cups natural crude kale
- ½ cup cubed shallots (could substitute onion)
- 2 cups cubed simmered butternut squash
- 10 eggs, beaten with a sprinkle of water
- ½ cup destroyed Parmigiano Reggiano cheddar
- Salt and pepper

Method:

- ✓ Preheat the broiler to 350 degrees. Broil ~1½-2 lb butternut squash for 35 minutes (cut squash down the middle longwise, scoop out seeds, serve squash daintily with olive oil, salt, and pepper, place cut side down on a foil-lined sheet. Heat 35 mins or until done. Should be possible early. You will not need the entirety of the squash for this dish).
- ✓ Beat eggs with a sprinkle of (a few tablespoons), mix in ½ cup parmesan cheddar put in a safe spot.
- ✓ Heat a broiler evidence skillet on medium heat, add 1 Tablespoon olive oil, add shallots and saute for 2-3 minutes. Add kale and keep on cooking for an extra 3 minutes or until kale is shriveled. Add roasted butternut squash. Serve vegetable combination with salt and pepper.

- ✓ Empty eggs into the skillet and delicately mix on more than one occasion to appropriate. Cook for 1-2 minutes or until eggs is set.
- ✓ Move to broiler for ~18 minutes or until cooked through.

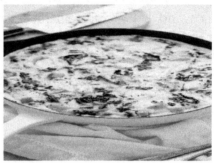

Recipe: 42

Sweet Potato Breakfast Hash

Sweet potato breakfast hash? Amazing. Thus basic. Grinding the sweet potatoes will save you an outing to the rec center (use the huge openings of a case grater), however from that point forward, you should simply broil them in a touch of margarine and sprinkle with salt and pepper. That's it. Just ground sweet potatoes, margarine, salt, and pepper. Avoid the salt if you are utilizing salted margarine.

Ingredients:

- 3 strips bacon
- 1/2 red pepper cubed
- 1/2 teaspoon stew powder
- 1/2 green pepper cubed
- 1/2 yellow onion cubed
- 1/2 teaspoon cumin
- 1/2 teaspoon dried oregano
- 1/2 teaspoon paprika
- 1/2 teaspoon garlic powder
- 3-4 huge eggs

- 1/2 teaspoon salt + more to taste
- 1/2 teaspoon black pepper
- 1 cup jalapeno and habanero jack cheddar approximately stuffed
- 1 - 1/2 pounds' sweet potatoes washed, stripped, and cubed into ½ inch 3D shapes

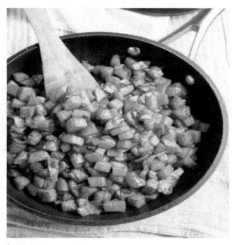

Method:

- ✓ Spot bacon in a chilly (stove safe) cast-iron skillet* in a solitary layer. Turn oven on to medium.
- ✓ Cook bacon until firm. Eliminate bacon from the dish, however, leave the bacon oil.
- ✓ Disintegrate bacon and put it in a safe spot.
- ✓ In a similar skillet, cook the potatoes in the bacon oil for 5 minutes until they begin to mollify.
- ✓ Include the green pepper, red pepper, onion, and flavors: stew powder, cumin, paprika, oregano, garlic powder, salt, and pepper.
- ✓ Cook until every one of the veggies is delicate, around 7-10 additional minutes.

Recipe: 43

Orange Shakshuka

Orange Shakshuka is a scrumptious variety of this much-cherished recipe, ideal for comfortable fall and cold weather months. It's a warm and fragrant blend of butternut squash, onion, orange chime pepper, vegetable stock, garlic, flavors, and spices. It's a basic, stewing blend with a couple of delicately poached eggs on top that you can appreciate.

Ingredients:

- Vegetable Broth
- Butternut Squash
- Onion and Garlic
- Orange Bell Pepper
- Flavors and Herbs
- Eggs

Method:

- ✓ Broil your butternut squash. Preheat your broiler to 400F, cut the squash fifty-fifty, and rub olive oil with a spot of salt and pepper. Cook face side down for around 40-45 minutes until the substance gets rich delicate.
- ✓ Sauté the aromatics. Mix the onion, chime pepper, and a little oil in an enormous search for gold minutes.
- ✓ In goes the flavors. Mix in the thyme, nutmeg, cumin, salt, and pepper until it's conhealthyated.
- ✓ Add the butternut squash. Scoop the fragile living creature and add it to the dish, alongside the vegetable stock. Separate the squash pieces and present to everything to a stew.
- ✓ Add the eggs. Make little wells with a spoon and break eggs into everyone. Then cover the container and let it cook for around 5 minutes, or until the eggs are however you would prefer.

✓ Topping and serve. Sprinkle your most loved microgreens, fresh thyme, cleaved parsley, or whichever spices you like. You can't turn out badly with any here!

Smoked Salmon Frittata

This Smoked Salmon Frittata is light, fleecy, and ideal for early lunch! Made with eggs, dill, tricks, smoked salmon, cream cheddar, red onion, and tomatoes, this tasty egg dish is consistently a group pleaser! Flavorful warm or cold.

Ingredients:

- 1 medium onion, cubed
- 12 extra-enormous eggs
- 1 tablespoon unsalted margarine
- 1 cup hefty cream
- 1/2 pound smoked salmon, cleaved
- 4 ounces'fresh goat cheddar, like Montrachet, disintegrated
- 3 scallions, slashed, white, and light green parts
- 1 teaspoon fit salt
- 3 tablespoons slashed fresh dill
- 1/2 teaspoon freshly ground black pepper

Method:

✓ Preheat the broiler to 350 degrees F.
✓ Saute the onion and margarine in a 10-inch stove evidence omelet skillet over medium-low heat until clear, around 5 minutes.
✓ In an enormous bowl, beat the eggs.
✓ Add the weighty cream, goat cheddar, smoked salmon, scallions, dill, salt, and pepper, and conhealthyate.
✓ Pour the combination over the onions and spot the omelet container in the focal point of the stove.

✓ Heat the frittata for around 50 minutes, until it puffs and a blade embedded in the center tells the truth. Serve hot straightforwardly from the dish.

Recipe: 45

Homemade Yogurt

There are various approaches to make natively constructed yogurt and if you read 10 distinct web journals about how to make custom-made yogurt, you're probably going to discover 10 unique varieties. Furthermore, that is because we've all discovered what works for us. There's no correct method to do it. What's more, fortunately, custom-made yogurt is darn excusing.

Ingredients:

- 1 gallon 2% milk
- 1 cup plain yogurt with dynamic societies

Method:

✓ Empty the milk into a pot and heat to the point of boiling, blending once in a while to forestall staying. Lessen heat and stew, around 10 minutes; don't allow it to bubble over.

✓ Eliminate pot from the heat and permit to sit for 30 to an hour.

✓ Plunge your finger into the milk occasionally to decide when you can leave your finger in the milk for 10 to 15 seconds without consuming it.

✓ Pour in the yogurt.

✓ Put the top on the pot and cautiously fold a cover over it. Spot the enclosed pot by a marginally warm where it will be undisturbed for 6 to 10 hours; short-term is ideal.

✓ Move to the fridge for stiffening.

Breakfast Egg Muffins

This Breakfast Egg Cups Recipe is the ideal breakfast in a hurry. Make them early, refrigerate or freeze them, and afterward heat them in the microwave when you are prepared to eat. They are high in protein and low in pretty much all the other things (carbs, sugar, and so on) This is a genuine energy food, my companions. Exactly what developing bodies need.

Ingredients:

- 2 spring onions
- 1 ringer pepper, red
- 6 eggs
- 1 modest bunch of spinach (or any green leaves)
- 1 tsp salt
- ½ cup cheddar (ground; other cheddar is fine as well)
- 4-5 sprinkles of hot sauce (or 1 tsp curry powder)

Method:

- ✓ Preheat the broiler to 200°C/390°F.
- ✓ Wash and dice the ringer pepper and onions. also, put them in a huge blending bowl.
- ✓ Wash the spinach, gently slash it and add it to the bowl too.
- ✓ Add the eggs and salt. Blend well. Professional tip – break the eggs independently before adding. That way if you get a dodgy one, it will not demolish the entire supper.
- ✓ Blend in the cheddar to the hitter.
- ✓ Add some hot sauce or curry powder.
- ✓ Oil the biscuit tin with oil and kitchen paper/preparing brush and empty the egg blend equally into the biscuit spaces.
- ✓ Pop the plate into the broiler for 20 minutes or until the tops are firm to the touch.

Walnut-Rosemary Crusted Salmon

The way to rolling out a healthy improvement is to set yourself up for progress, and it's imperative to perceive what your body needs to roll out those improvements occur. Investigate your sustenance and how you are preparing your nourishment for the week. The correct decisions in food will fuel your body, at last improving your wellbeing, mindset, rest, and perhaps a lot more parts of your regular daily existence.

Begin taking a gander at what the food you're devouring has to bring to the table. Salmon and pecans are both incredible wellsprings of omega-3 unsaturated fats. Pair this simple salmon recipe with a basic salad and a side of cooked potatoes or quinoa.

Ingredients:

- 1 clove garlic, minced
- 2 teaspoons Dijon mustard
- 1/4 teaspoon lemon zing
- 1 teaspoon cleaved fresh rosemary
- 1 teaspoon lemon juice
- 1/2 teaspoon nectar
- 1/4 teaspoon squashed red pepper
- 1/2 teaspoon genuine salt
- 3 tablespoons finely cleaved pecans
- 3 tablespoons panko breadcrumbs
- Olive oil cooking shower
- 1 teaspoon extra-virgin olive oil
- (1 pound) skinless salmon filet, fresh or frozen

Method:

- ✓ Preheat broiler to 425 degrees F. Line a huge rimmed preparing sheet with material paper.

- ✓ Join mustard, garlic, lemon zing, lemon juice, rosemary, nectar, salt, and squashed red pepper in a little bowl.
- ✓ Conhealthyate panko, pecans, and oil in another little bowl.
- ✓ Spot salmon on the readied heating sheet.
- ✓ Spread the mustard combination over the fish and sprinkle with the panko blend, squeezing to follow. Delicately cover with a cooking shower.
- ✓ Heat until the fish chips effectively with a fork, around 8 to 12 minutes, contingent upon thickness.
- ✓ Sprinkle with parsley and present with lemon wedges, whenever wanted.

Easy Oatmeal Recipe

It's one of the most effortless (and quickest) quality suppers you can make. Appreciate a fundamental bowl of cereal (nothing amiss with that), or get innovative with perpetual sweet and exquisite flavor choices. You can't beat how straightforward a bowl of oats is to modify. You can decide to serve it plain with a sprinkle of milk or dress it up with your number one garnishes.

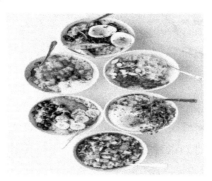

Ingredients:

- Moved Oats
- Water or Milk
- Salt
- Garnishes

Method:

- ✓ Bubble water. In a little pot, heat the water or milk and salt to the point of boiling over medium-high heat.
- ✓ Cook the oats. Mix in the oats then diminishes the heat to medium-low. Allow it to stew for around 5 minutes to allow the fluid to ingest, while blending every so often.
- ✓ Top and serve. Add delightful garnishes, a sprinkle of milk if you'd like, and appreciate.

Best Hummus Recipe

The best hummus is delectably velvety, yet by one way or another light and cushioned. It's wonderfully smooth and whirled, and asking to be gathered up onto a wedge of pita bread. It's nutty and tart, on account of the tahini, with notes of splendid, fresh lemon and smooth garlic.

Ingredients:

- 2 garlic cloves
- 1/2 cup tahini
- 2 lemons, squeezed
- 1/4 cup olive oil
- 1 tsp cumin
- 1/2 tsp salt
- 1/3 cup chickpea fluid, or more, depending on the situation
- 30 oz canned chickpeas (garbanzo beans), depleted with fluid saved (I use two 15oz jars)

Method:

- ✓ Add every one of the ingredients to your Vitamix or powerful blender and secure the cover. Eliminate the cover cap and addition the alter.
- ✓ Turn the blender on high for 30 seconds (or more for a creamier surface) and use the alter to drive the hummus into the sharp edges. Add more chickpea fluid (aquafaba), whenever wanted, for a milder hummus.
- ✓ Add the hummus to a serving plate and embellishment with olive oil, paprika, and fresh parsley.

Recipe: 50

Best Lentil Soup

Lentil soup is an exemplary veggie-lover soup recipe. It's generous, healthy, superbly loading up (with plant-based protein), and warming on those chilly, frigid days. While there are numerous varieties of lentil soup, you can't turn out badly with a straightforward, tasty Mediterranean adaptation.

Ingredients:

- 1 medium onion, slashed
- 4 garlic cloves, minced
- 2 tablespoons coconut oil
- 3 tablespoons minced ginger
- ¼ teaspoon squashed red pepper drops, more to taste
- 1 tablespoon gentle curry powder
- 1 (28-ounce) can fire simmered cubed tomatoes
- 1 cup dried French green lentils, flushed and depleted
- 1 (14-ounce) can of full-fat coconut milk
- 2½ cups water
- ½ teaspoon ocean salt, more to taste
- ½ cup cubed cilantro
- Freshly ground black pepper
- 2 tablespoons fresh lime juice

Method:

- ✓ Heat the oil in a huge pot over medium heat. Add the onion and a touch of salt and cook until delicate and daintily sautéed around the edges, 8 to 10 minutes, diminishing the heat to low on a case by case basis.
- ✓ With the heat on low, add the garlic, ginger, curry powder, and red pepper pieces and cook, mixing, until fragrant, around 2 minutes.
- ✓ Add the tomatoes, lentils, water, coconut milk, ½ teaspoon salt, and a few drudgeries of black pepper. Heat to the point of boiling, cover, and decrease to a stew, blending just infrequently, until the lentils are delicate, 25 to 35 minutes. If your soup is excessively thick, mix in 1/2 to 1 cup more water to arrive at your ideal consistency.

Mix in the cilantro and lime juice. Serve to taste with salt and pepper and serve.

Lentil Salad with Cucumber

Lentil Salad Recipe with Cucumber is a straightforward and reviving side dish or light lunch. I'll tell you the best way to cook healthy dried lentils so they're delicate, not soft. This Mediterranean Lentil Salad is a generous salad that is ideal for lunch, a side dish, or even a veggie-lover primary dish. Rich in cucumbers, tomatoes, olives, feta, and protein pressed lentils. You'll cherish the flavors and surfaces in this healthy salad.

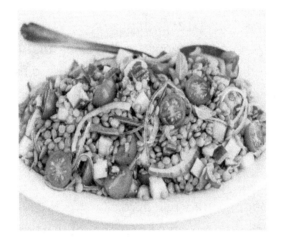

Ingredients:

- Cucumber, stripped and cubed (1 cup)
- Brown colored or green lentils (1 cup)
- Tomato, cubed (1 cup)
- Garlic, finely slashed (1 clove)
- Olives slashed (1 tbsp.)
- Balsamic vinegar (1/4 cup)
- Orange or red pepper, cubed (1 cup)
- Fresh basil slashed (1 tbsp.)

Method:

- ✓ Clean the lentils to ensure they have no stones and fill an enormous pot of water.
- ✓ Bubble delicately for 20 minutes or until delicate. Strain and let cool on a plate in the fridge.
- ✓ In a huge bowl, blend the lentils in with the leftover ingredients. Serve with salt and pepper.
- ✓ Serve the plate of mixed greens with cold.

Recipe: 52

Chicken & Spinach Skillet Pasta with Lemon & Parmesan

I have an arrangement for supper this evening that includes a basic rundown of ingredients including pasta, chicken, and fresh spinach. It's made across the board skillet and it will be on your table in around 30 minutes. This Chicken and Spinach Skillet Pasta is the thing that I call a strong arrangement.

Ingredients:

- 2 tablespoons extra-virgin olive oil
- 8-ounce gluten-free penne pasta or entire wheat penne pasta
- ½ teaspoon salt
- ¼ teaspoon ground pepper
- 10 cups hacked fresh spinach
- ½ cup dry white wine
- 4 cloves garlic, minced
- Squeeze and zing of 1 lemon
- 4 tablespoons ground Parmesan cheddar, separated
- 1 pound boneless, skinless chicken bosom or thighs, managed, if fundamental, and cut into scaled-down pieces

Method:

- ✓ Cook pasta as per bundle bearings. Filter and put in a safe spot.
- ✓ In the interim, heat oil in a huge high-sided skillet over medium-high heat. Add chicken, salt, and pepper; cook, mixing at times until just cooked through, 5 to 7 minutes.
- ✓ Add garlic and cook, blending, until fragrant, around 1 moment. Mix in wine, lemon squeeze, and zing; bring to a stew.
- ✓ Eliminate from heat. Mix in spinach and the cooked pasta.
- ✓ Cover and let remain until the spinach is simply shriveled.
- ✓ Split between 4 plates and top each presenting with 1 tablespoon Parmesan.

Recipe: 53

Baked Tuna Meatballs

The good food in a state of the ball. If you need to enhance the protein base and healthy unsaturated fats, these healthy and fit fish balls will do it simple peasy. You can set them up rapidly, effectively, and in a healthy way.

You can plan heated fish balls for instance with flavorful fish. It contains a great deal of omega-3 unsaturated fats, which effects affect the state of the heart, mind, and eyes and it is battling persistent aggravation. f

Anyhow, if you lean toward a higher fat substance and you simply love finely rich salmon, you will like salmon fish balls also. Subsequently, use either fish or salmon in the recipe, the two renditions are astoundingly delectable.

Ingredients:

- 20g (0.7oz) oats (I suggest these)
- 250g (8.8oz) fish in the water (I suggest this one)
- 1 egg
- ground black pepper
- ocean salt (I suggest this one)
- garlic powder

Method:

- ✓ Granulate or mix oats until fine.
- ✓ In a bowl, blend oats in with depleted fish, egg, and flavors to taste.
- ✓ Shape the mixture into balls and spot them onto a heating sheet fixed with material paper.
- ✓ Prepare the balls at 180 degrees Celsius (350 °F) for 20 minutes.
- ✓ Serve balls warm – ideally with yogurt, dill, or tomato

Recipe: 54

Dijon Baked Salmon

This Dijon salmon recipe is a family top pick. It's succulent, delicate, and simple to make. We make baked salmon consistently and love it since it's simple, simple, and very brisk. A portion of our famous baked salmon recipes are nectar lemon baked salmon in foil, broiler baked salmon with olives and escapades, and simple baked salmon filet with lemon. This Dijon salmon recipe is another most loved recipe of our own that is so tasty because of Dijon mustard and fresh dill.

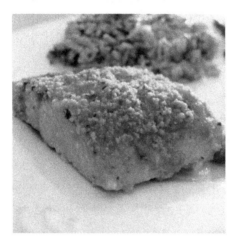

Ingredients:

- 3 tablespoons Dijon mustard
- ¼ cup spread softened
- 1 ½ tablespoon nectar
- ¼ cup finely hacked walnuts
- ¼ cup dry bread pieces
- 4 teaspoons hacked fresh parsley
- salt and pepper to taste
- (4 ounces) filets of salmon
- 1 lemon, to decorate

Method:

- ✓ Preheat the broiler to 400 degrees F.
- ✓ In a little bowl, mix margarine, mustard, and nectar.
- ✓ In another bowl, combine as one bread piece, walnuts, and parsley.
- ✓ Brush every salmon filet delicately with a nectar mustard combination, and sprinkle the highest points of the filets with the bread scrap blend.
- ✓ Prepare salmon for 12 to 15 minutes on the prebaked stove, or until it chips effectively with a fork.
- ✓ Serve with salt and pepper, and embellish with a wedge of lemon.

Recipe: 55

Roasted Branzino with Citrus Pesto

Roasted branzino filets are finished off with citrus pesto and an assortment of occasional citrus cuts. It's a basic, solid, and flavorful fish recipe. Branzino is a tasty, sensitive, and gentle white fish that passes by numerous names. In Italy, it's branzino. In different pieces of the world, it very well might be also called European seabass, Mediterranean seabass, Spingola, loup de Mer, ocean dace, lubina, or robalo.

Ingredients:

- 6 branzino filets
- 1 lemon, zested, and squeezed
- salt and pepper, to taste
- 2 tbsp olive oil
- 1/4 cup olive oil
- 1 clove garlic
- 1/3 cup pine nuts, toasted
- 1 orange, zested and squeezed
- salt and pepper, to taste
- 1 lemon, cut
- 2 oranges, cut
- 1 cup fresh basil leaves, decently pressed

Method:

- ✓ Preheat the stove to 350 degrees Fahrenheit.
- ✓ Spot the branzino filets on a material-lined preparing plate. Softly cover the fillets in olive oil and sprinkle with salt and pepper. Cook for 12 minutes, or until cooked through.
- ✓ While the branzino is cooking, delicately toast the pine nuts in a dish in the oven. Add the toasted pine nuts alongside the leftover citrus pesto ingredients to a food processor and heartbeat a few times until you have pesto.
- ✓ Cut the lemon and oranges for the top topping with a mandoline and put in a safe spot
- ✓ At the point when the branzino is cooked through, place it on a serving platter and top each filet with the citrus pesto and a couple of citrus cuts.

Best Baked Cod

This baked cod is my simple and idiot-proof recipe for totally flaky fish, without fail. A basic rich and garlicky spice besting change simple cod filets into a light and sound weeknight dish.

Ingredients:

- ½2 tablespoons spread
- ½ lemon, squeezed
- 1 tablespoon hacked green onion
- 1 tablespoon hacked fresh parsley
- ¼ cup dry white wine
- 1 pound thick-cut cod midsection
- 1 lemon, cut into wedges
- sleeve rich round wafers, squashed
- 2 tablespoons spread

Method:

- ✓ Preheat stove to 200 degrees C.
- ✓ Spot 2 tablespoons spread in a microwave-safe bowl; liquefy in the microwave on high, around 30 seconds. Mix rich round saltines into dissolved margarine.
- ✓ Spot staying 2 tablespoons margarine in a 7x11-inch preparing dish. Dissolve in the prebaked broiler, 1 to 3 minutes. Eliminate dish from broiler.
- ✓ Coat the two sides of cod in liquefied margarine in the preparing dish.
- ✓ Heat cod in the prebaked broiler for 10 minutes. Eliminate from broiler; top with lemon juice, wine, and saltine blend. Spot back in the broiler and prepare until fish is black and pieces effectively with a fork, around 10 additional minutes.
- ✓ Baked cod with parsley and green onion. Present with lemon wedges.

Barbunya Pilaki

Barbunya Pilaki could be known as the Turkish variant of baked beans. Here, cranberry beans are cooked with tasty vegetables giving a light and invigorating option in contrast to conventional, intensely sauced baked beans. Serve this make-ahead dish warm or cold at your spring outing or summer grill.

Ingredients:

- 1 Tbsp olive oil
- 2 garlic cloves, minced
- 1 Tbsp tomato glue
- ½ tsp salt
- 1 tsp sugar
- ¼ tsp ground black pepper
- 1 – 1 ½ c water
- Fresh parsley and lemon wedges
- 2 carrots, cubed
- 2 huge tomatoes, cubed, or 1 (14oz can) cubed tomatoes, with juices
- 1 onion, cubed
- 1 c dried borlotti or pinto beans, splashed for the time being

Method:

- ✓ Add splashed and depleted beans to a huge pan and cover with one inch of water.
- ✓ Heat the beans to the point of boiling and decrease the heat to medium-low. Stew the beans until simply delicate, 20-30 minutes.
- ✓ In an enormous skillet, heat olive oil. Add the onion and garlic. Sauté for 2-3 minutes over medium heat, until delicate.
- ✓ Add the carrots and sauté for 5 min. Add the tomatoes, tomato glue, sugar, salt, and pepper. Blend well.
- ✓ Add the cooked, depleted beans and freshwater (utilize 1 ½ c of water if utilizing fresh tomatoes or 1 c of water if utilizing canned tomatoes with juices).
- ✓ Blend well and stew, revealed over medium-low heat, until the majority of the fluid has vanished, 30 minutes, mixing once in a while.
- ✓ The dish can be served promptly or refrigerated and served cold.
- ✓ To serve, embellish beans with slashed fresh parsley and lemon cut

Recipe: 58

Mediterranean Chickpea Salad

This simple Mediterranean chickpea salad is mixed with flavor on account of a stacking aiding of fresh spices with a garlicky lemon dressing that ups the mash from red ringer pepper, celery, and red onion for a basic side dish or ingredient for greens.

Chickpea salad has been one of my go-to snacks for quite a long time. With class kickoff serve close to the corner, I thought I'd share my #1 chickpea salad recipe with every one of you! In light of the protein from the chickpeas, it's generous enough to be a supper all alone, however, it can likewise serve as a sound side dish.

Ingredients:

Salad:

- 1 English cucumber cubed
- 30 ounces canned chickpeas depleted and washed
- 1 green chime pepper cubed
- 1/2 cup disintegrated feta
- 1 little red onion meagerly cut
- 1/2 cup cut kalamata olives
- 2 tablespoons freshly cleaved basil
- 1-16 ounces red grape or cherry tomatoes divided or quartered
- 2 tablespoons freshly cleaved mint

Dressing:

- 2 tablespoons nectar
- 3 tablespoons additional virgin olive oil
- 2 tablespoons lemon juice
- 2 tablespoons white wine vinegar
- 1/4 teaspoon salt
- 1/4 teaspoon black pepper

Method:

- ✓ In a huge blending bowl, put together feta, chickpeas, tomato, cucumber, chime pepper, basil, red onion, olives, and mint.
- ✓ For the dressing, empty nectar into a microwave-safe blending bowl. Microwave 10-15 seconds to liquify nectar. Race in olive oil, lemon juice, vinegar, salt, and pepper.
- ✓ Pour dressing over chickpea salad. Put to consolidate. Refrigerate until baked to serve.

Recipe: 59

Tuna Salad

Ideal for tuna salad sandwiches or smooth fish dissolves with some coleslaw as an afterthought! Prepare a salad or sandwiches or even scoop it into a large portion of avocado for an extravagant (and low carb) dish. Any can or container of fish will work in a sandwich. Simply ensure you channel the water or oil before blending in with the elements for tuna salad.

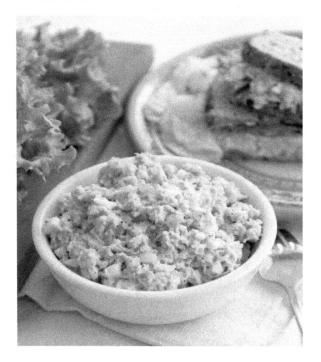

Ingredients:

- Two 6-ounce jars of white meat fish pressed in water, depleted
- 1 teaspoon minced level leaf parsley
- 2 tablespoons minced celery
- 1/3 cup arranged mayonnaise
- Freshly ground black pepper
- 1 tablespoon entire grain mustard
- Freshly crushed lemon juice (discretionary)
- 2 tablespoons minced red onion, absorbed virus water for 5 minutes, and depleted

Method:

- ✓ In a little blending, the bowl separates the fish with a fork.
- ✓ Put with celery, onion, and parsley.
- ✓ Add the mayonnaise, mustard and serve with pepper, to taste.
- ✓ Mix to consolidate.
- ✓ Add lemon juice, to taste, if utilizing.

Salmon Patties

Salmon Patties, produced using wild got canned salmon, are simple to make supper time top pick in our home and are the best salmon cake recipe ever. It has likewise consistently been my family's #1 supper.

Ingredients:

- 1 cup Panko breadcrumbs
- 1 little onion (or 1/2 huge), ground
- 1 garlic, minced
- 1/4 tsp each salt and pepper
- 1/3 cup fresh dill, generally cleaved (or 1 tsp dried spices of decision)
- 2 eggs
- 2 shallots/scallions/green onions, finely cut
- 1/2 cup parmesan, ground or destroyed
- 400 g/14 oz cooked fresh salmon OR canned red or pink salmon, depleted

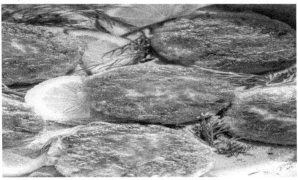

Method:

- ✓ Preheat stove to 220C/430F norm (200C fan)
- ✓ Spot breadcrumbs in a bowl. Mesh over the onion, including juices.

- ✓ Blend onion into breadcrumbs, guaranteeing all breadcrumbs are doused.
- ✓ Add remaining ingredients aside from salmon.
- ✓ Blend well.
- ✓ Add salmon. Mix through delicately, leaving drops of salmon (instead of energetically blending salmon into little pieces).
- ✓ Gather up 1/4 cup combination.
- ✓ Structure round patties about 1.5 cm/2/3" thick and put in a safe spot.
- ✓ Sprinkle oil all over the plate.
- ✓ Spot in the stove for 2 minutes until hot - oil will spread over the plate.
- ✓ Slant plate to spread if necessary.
- ✓ Spot patties on the plate - DO NOT press down (makes them stick on the plate). Shower surface with oil splash.
- ✓ Prepare 15 minutes. Flip, shower surface with oil splash, heat 5 minutes.
- ✓ Present with sharp cream or yogurt as an afterthought for plunging/dolloping, and extra fresh dill whenever wanted.
- ✓ I served mine with cauliflower puree and Yogurt Slaw - sound side alternatives!

Lemon Shrimp Pasta

This smooth lemon shrimp pasta recipe is sufficiently simple to make on a weeknight and adequately amazing to serve at an evening gathering. This velvety shrimp pasta recipe is one of my top choices. Now and again a rich pasta is the only thing that will do.

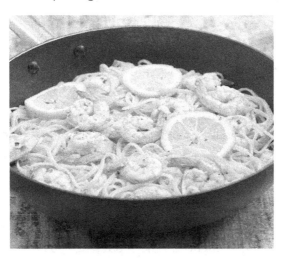

Ingredients:

- 1-pound shrimp (I utilized 31-40 check size) stripped and defrosted
- 8-ounce pasta (I utilized spaghetti)
- 3 tablespoons spread
- 1 cup substantial/whipping cream
- 6 cloves garlic minced
- 1/2 cup dry white wine
- 2 teaspoons flour
- 1 cup freshly ground parmesan cheddar
- 2 runs of Italian flavoring
- Salt and pepper to taste
- Hacked parsley (discretionary)
- Zing and juice of one lemon (around 2 tbsp lemon juice)

Method:

- ✓ Heat an enormous, all-around salted pot of water for the pasta. Cook still somewhat firm as coordinated.
- ✓ Then, add the spread, lemon zing and lemon juice, minced garlic, white wine, cream, and Italian flavoring to a skillet over medium-high heat.
- ✓ Allow the sauce to rise for 5 minutes.
- ✓ Bit by bit add the flour to the sauce, mixing/beating continually to guarantee the sauce is smooth.
- ✓ Mix in the parmesan cheddar.
- ✓ Keep on stewing the sauce on medium heat for an extra 5 minutes, blending as often as possible. The sauce ought to be recognizably thickened at this point. If not, keep stewing it for a couple of more minutes.
- ✓ Add shrimp and keep on cooking for an extra 5 minutes until sauce is thickened as wanted and shrimp are cooked.
- ✓ Channel the spaghetti, then put the pasta with the sauce. Sprinkle with fresh parsley. Serve right away.

Conclusion:

You may have seen that these Mediterranean Diet Recipes use extra virgin olive oil. t s because extra virgin olive oil is produced using the absolute first squeezing of the olives, and as an outcome contains the most elevated levels of antioxidants. The Mediterranean Diet is renowned for being a rich source of antioxidants, which are essential for good health and cleaning up risky free revolutionaries.

I hope you will appreciate these Mediterranean Diet Recipes.

What to cook when you have a lot of leftover vegetables in your fridge? One idea is to make a frittata and in particular, a spinach, mushroom, feta and tomato frittata. It's that perfect brunch or lunch recipe that is fast, delicious and easy on the budget.